T0163702

The Little Book of
MEDICAL QUOTES

Inspiring Thoughts in Medicine

Daniel McMahon, MD

tfm Publishing Limited, Castle Hill Barns, Harley, Shrewsbury, SY5 6LX, UK
Tel: +44 (0)1952 510061; Fax: +44 (0)1952 510192
E-mail: info@tfmpublishing.com; Web site: www.tfmpublishing.com

Editing, design & typesetting: Nikki Bramhill BSc Hons Dip Law
Cover image © Comstock Inc., www.comstock.com

First edition:	© 2020
Hardback	ISBN: 978-1-910079-83-6
ePub	ISBN: 978-1-910079-84-3
Mobi	ISBN: 978-1-910079-85-0
Web pdf	ISBN: 978-1-910079-86-7

Printed by Gutenberg Press Ltd., Gudja Road, Tarxien, GXQ 2902, Malta
Tel: +356 2398 2201; Fax: +356 2398 2290
E-mail: info@gutenberg.com.mt; Web site: www.gutenberg.com.mt

Contents

PART I THE PRACTICE OF PHYSICK

PART II PILLARS OF TIMELESS WISDOM FOR CLINICAL PRACTICE

PART III PHILOSOPHIC INSPIRATION & WORDS TO LIVE BY

PART IV THE ROAD AHEAD

Introduction

You have chosen the most fascinating and dynamic profession
there is, a profession with the highest potential for greatness,
since the physician's daily work is wrapped up in the subtle web
of history. Your labors are linked with those of your colleagues
who preceded you in history, and those who are now working
all over the world. It is this spiritual unity with our colleagues of
all periods and all countries that has made medicine so universal
and eternal. For this reason we must study and try to imitate the
lives of the "Great Doctors" of history.

Félix Martí-Ibáñez
(1911-1972; Spanish-American physician)

The rich history of medicine is a perpetually evolving canvas that over the course of multiple millennia continues to be adorned with a bold palate of colors and courageous brushstrokes. Through examination of the written and spoken word, we are able to peel away the centuries-old layers of paint enameled upon the dynamic canvas of medical history and examine the vast progress that has occurred as time dutifully marches forward. While the landscapes portrayed may change, the thematic truths, ideals, and fundamental tenets ubiquitous to the practice of compassionate and sound medical care remain an everlastingly vibrant focal point that has never faded nor been painted over.

The historic practice of medicine, among primitive civilizations and ancient empires, was a seemingly magical discipline loosely based upon rudimentary scientific principles and theories once widely accepted in the era of antiquity. Thomas Sydenham, a 17th century English physician noted, "As no man can say who it was that first invented the use of clothes and houses against the inclemency of the weather, so also can no investigator point out the origin of medicine — mysterious as the source of the Nile." In stark contrast to the arcane healthcare practices of the antediluvian era, the contemporary practice of medicine is woven directly into the fabric of our society and culture with roots firmly embedded in cutting-edge science and technology. Although modern-day healthcare practices and scientific advancements continue to briskly distance themselves from antiquated theories such as humorism, medicine nevertheless endures as a timeless edifice with steadfast ties to the ageless traditions of philosophy and art.

This collection of quotations, cast across thousands of years, is comprised of inspirational thoughts and universal ideals that remain enduringly coupled to the art, science, and philosophy of medical practice. These selected quotes include a wide breadth of keen observations and aphorisms linked to the history, grounding principles, and fundamental theories of medicine spanning multiple millennia from the ancient epochs to the contemporary era. These thoughts are drawn from past generations of legendary physicians and intrepid explorers of medical science as well as distinguished anatomists, physiologists, and philosophers. Additionally, you will find the following chapters to be polished with a variety of engaging medical quotes from scholarly figures throughout history including writers, artists, and statesmen.

A particularly unique aspect of this collection, complementing the primary theme of medicine, is the addition of numerous motivational quotes which substantively address the pursuit of success in medical practice as well as in actualizing personal goals and dreams. While a number of these quotations originate from influential persons throughout history that may not be inherently involved in medicine, I believe we can draw tremendous insight from these inspiring truisms. These quotations adeptly liven the discourse of medicine and healing through the concomitant examination of many fascinating thoughts related to the quest to achieve success and value.

As I began to research this collection of quotations, I enthusiastically uncovered an immensely intriguing level of candor that is directly applicable to the contemporary practice of medicine. As a result, I felt a calling to spread these beautiful thoughts, from many truly beautiful minds throughout history, so we may all learn and grow from their wisdom. Consider these quotations a daily dose of inspiration regardless of the particular discipline or specialty of medicine you have chosen to pursue.

In the following pages you will ponder logical precepts, universal truths, and cogent words of guidance from ancient physicians and philosophers such as Hippocrates, Aristotle, and Socrates. You will be offered sage counsel from famed giants of *medical history including Armand Trousseau, Sir William Osler, Michael E. DeBakey, and many others. Hear poignant thoughts that have been bestowed upon us from world-renowned medical scientists who courageously plied the staggering depths of uncharted scientific waters such as Claude Bernard, Jonas Salk, and Marie Curie. In doing so, these brave pioneers profoundly brought to light extraordinary new discoveries that radically advanced the field of medicine. Allow yourself to be captivated by enlightening tenets delivered from the most celebrated Renaissance men, scientists, and innovators known in the history of the world including Leonardo da Vinci, Sir Isaac Newton, and Albert Einstein.*

A majority of the historic figures quoted in the following chapters will be recognized as household names; however, other names may seem a bit more obscure. Compiling these quotations from both widely known as well as less widely recognized contributors, who are nonetheless irrevocably important to the genre of medical and surgical history, has proven to be an unbelievably rich and informative experience.

Despite language that is sometimes written in verbiage and prose echoing from centuries past, this is a common language that we all as medical professionals can relate to. Whether you are a house officer, junior attending, or seasoned staff, these quotes were written for you and they will undoubtedly speak to you. I believe this collection is especially poignant for medical trainees who have arrived at a crucial inflection point in their early careers and professional development. These quotations have the capacity to bring into clear focus the fundamentals and principles that are illustrative of sound medical practice, empathetic patient care, and humble professionalism.

In a medical world that has become overwhelming inundated with convoluted electronic health records and complex diagnostic services, we must not forget these simple yet profound truths. Furthermore, we must remember to employ the guidance contained therein at the most fundamental levels of medical practice. These thoughts are not complex; however, they are nevertheless cognitively stimulating and at times they are refreshingly witty and humorous. Allow these time-tested precepts to convey a modicum of simplicity, richness, and brightness upon your complex world.

While some of these ideals may seem archaic, they certainly continue to hold true in the contemporary sphere of medicine and surgery. These quotations remain resilient to the weathering effects of the dynamic world evolving around us *despite centuries and millennia that have elapsed in some cases. The luster, shine, and crisply resounding ring and tone of these thoughts have not in the least been dulled nor tarnished by the burgeoning influences of time. Although trends, fads, and fashions ebb and flow in the discipline of medicine, like everything else, these truths never lose their application or appeal. Nor should they.*

Heed the advice and experience of those who have come before us. In doing so, become an astute student of medical, philosophic, and scientific history. Allow the knowledge and wisdom bestowed upon us from these colossal figures of history to mentor your path forward as a well-rounded, driven, and humble practitioner. As per the wise words of Sir Isaac Newton, "I can see so far because I stood on the shoulders of giants."

Beginning your day with an optimistic quotation can at times have a profound effect upon how you approach your duties and your patients. It is my sincere hope that these thoughts, taken in daily doses or perused in larger sections as desired, will manifest themselves as a means to starting your day on the right foot and invigorate your mind and body to carry out the calling of a medical professional with excellence. Overall, I have tried with much restraint to keep my own

commentary for each chapter to a minimum so the reader may
draw his or her own personal parallels and introspective
musings. I hope you gain as much personal motivation,
inspiration, and insight from these thoughts as I have
throughout the process of assembling this collection. Enjoy!

Daniel McMahon, MD

Medicine is the one place where all the show is stripped of
the human drama. You, as doctors, will be in a position to see
the human race stark naked — not only physically, but
mentally and morally as well.

Martin H. Fischer
(1879-1962; German-American physician & author)

About the
author

Daniel McMahon is a native of Fairhope, Alabama. He received an undergraduate degree in biology from the University of Alabama and was awarded a Navy Health Professions Scholarship to complete his Doctor of Medicine training at the University of Alabama School of Medicine. Following medical school he completed general surgery internship training at the Naval Medical Center Portsmouth, Virginia, prior to a course of aerospace medical and flight training at the Naval Aerospace Medical Institute in Pensacola, Florida, where he was designated a naval flight surgeon.

After flight surgery training he completed a two-year operational flight surgery tour while based in Lemoore, California, with Carrier Air Wing Eleven. During this tour, he embarked aboard the aircraft carrier, USS Nimitz, in support of carrier strike group exercises and fleet operations. He was also deployed with Carrier Air Wing Fourteen, aboard USS Ronald Reagan, in support of Operation Enduring Freedom and Operation Iraqi Freedom. Following his flight surgery tour, he went on to complete general surgery residency training at the Naval Medical Center Portsmouth, Virginia. At the conclusion of his formal surgical training he completed a two-year overseas tour as a staff general surgeon at the Naval Hospital Yokosuka, Japan, where he served as the Department Head for the Department of General Surgery. Additionally, during this overseas tour he was deployed as Officer-In-Charge of an austere expeditionary surgical team in support of Naval Special Operations forces.

Shortly after this overseas tour of duty he was deployed to Afghanistan where he served as a forward trauma surgeon in support of Operation Freedom's Sentinel and the Resolute Support Mission. Following this deployment, he returned to the Naval Hospital Pensacola, Florida, where he currently serves as a staff general surgeon.

He is a member of the American College of Surgeons as well as the Excelsior Surgical Society and is an Assistant Professor of Surgery with the Uniformed Services University of Health Sciences. He lives in Mobile, Alabama, with his wife Aurelia and his two children Benton and Aurelia Marie, where he enjoys hunting, fishing, and spending time with friends and family.

Dedication

The trained nurse has become one of the great blessings of humanity, taking a place beside the physician and the priest.

Sir William Osler
(1849-1919; Canadian physician)

I would like to offer my most sincere thanks and gratitude to all of the nurses, physician's assistants, nurse practitioners, surgical assistants, patient care technicians, healthcare staff, office staff, and facilities staff that we as physicians have the privilege to serve alongside as we carry out the wonderful profession we have been trained to practice. Without the compassion and empathy of these truly selfless and wonderful teammates we would never succeed in the art of healing. You all consistently and tirelessly make positive, ineffaceable, and meaningful impacts upon the lives of our patients and your dedication does not go unnoticed. Thank you!

Part I

THE PRACTICE OF PHYSICK

Whatever State of the Human Body doth disorder the
Vital, the Natural, or even the Animal Functions of the
same is called a Disease. And that part of the Science or
Art of Physick, which teacheth how to find out the
Disease actually afflicting the Patient, and how to cure
the same, is called The Practice of Physick. A Cure is
the Changing of a Disease into Health.

Herman Boerhaave
(1668-1738; Dutch botanist,
chemist, & physician)

Chapter 1

A noble & altruistic calling

No greater opportunity, responsibility, or obligation can fall to the lot of a human being than to become a physician. In the care of the suffering he needs technical skill, scientific knowledge, and human understanding. He who uses these with courage, with humility, and with wisdom will provide a unique service for his fellow man, and will build an enduring edifice of character within himself. The physician should ask of his destiny no more than this; he should be content with no less.

Tinsley R. Harrison
(1900-1978; American physician)

3

● *As a physician you provide a noble and altruistic service to the fellow citizens of your communities, metropolitans, and perhaps even farther abroad on a global level. Take great pride in this service you provide. Although we all get lost in the minutiae of our day-to-day professional and personal lives, take a moment to reflect upon the privilege we have been granted as physicians to impart a healing influence upon the patients we are entrusted to care for. Endeavor to maintain an unwavering appreciation for the art and science of medicine and surgery as well as an unrelenting drive to continue carrying out the responsibilities and obligations of our timeless profession with empathy, passion, and dedication that each and every one of our patients are deserving of.*

DM

First, it must be a pleasure to study the human body the most miraculous masterpiece of nature and to learn about the smallest vessel and the smallest fiber. But second and most important, the medical profession gives the opportunity to alleviate the troubles of the body, to ease the pain, to console a person who is in distress, and to lighten the hour of death of many a sufferer.

Rudolph Virchow
(1821-1902; German physician)

✦ There are some arts which to those that possess them are painful, but to those that use them are helpful, a common good to laymen, but to those that practise them grievous. Of such arts there is one which the Greeks call medicine. For the medical man sees terrible sights, touches unpleasant things, and the misfortunes of others bring a harvest of sorrows that are peculiarly his; but the sick by means of the art rid themselves of the worst of evils, disease, suffering, pain and death.

Hippocrates
(460 BC-370 BC; Greek physician)

✦ The practice of medicine will be very much as you make it — to one a worry, a care, a perpetual annoyance; to another, a daily job and a life of as much happiness and usefulness as can well fall to the lot of man, because it is a life of self-sacrifice and of countless opportunities to comfort and help the weak-hearted, and to raise up those that fall.

Sir William Osler
(1849-1919; Canadian physician)

✦ If we had nothing but pecuniary rewards and worldly honours to look to, our profession would not be one to be desired. But in its practice you will find it to be attended with peculiar privileges, second to none in intense interest and pure pleasures. It is our proud office to tend the fleshly tabernacle of the immortal spirit, and our path, rightly followed, will be guided by unfettered truth and love unfeigned. In the pursuit of this noble and holy calling I wish you all God-speed.

Joseph Lister
(1827-1912; British surgeon)

✦ An inquiring, analytical mind; an unquenchable thirst for new knowledge; and a heartfelt compassion for the ailing — these are prominent traits among the committed clinicians who have preserved the passion for medicine.

Michael E. DeBakey
(1908-2008; American cardiovascular surgeon)

✦ But nothing is more estimable than a physician who, having studied nature from his youth, knows the properties of the human body, the diseases which assail it, the remedies which will benefit it, exercises his art with caution, and pays equal attention to the rich and the poor.

Francois-Marie Arouet, known by his nom de plume, Voltaire (1694-1778; French writer & philosopher)

✦ In our daily patients we witness human nature in the raw — fear, despair, courage, understanding, hope, resignation, heroism. If alert, we can detect new problems to solve, new paths to investigate.

Joseph Murray (1919-2012; American surgeon)

✦ Only those who regard healing as the ultimate goal of their efforts can, therefore, be designated as physicians.

Rudolph Virchow (1821-1902; German physician)

✦ All knowledge attains its ethical value and its human significance only by the human sense with which it is employed. Only a good man can be a great physician.

Hermann Nothnagel
(1841-1905; German physician)

✦ The true physician has a Shakespearean breadth of interest in the wise and the foolish, the proud and the humble, the stoic hero and the whining rouge. He cares for people.

Tinsley R. Harrison
(1900-1978; American physician)

✦ The practice of medicine is an art, not a trade; a calling, not a business; a calling in which your heart will be exercised equally with your head. Often the best part of your work will have nothing to do with potions and powders, but with the exercise of an influence of the strong upon the weak, of the righteous upon the wicked, of the wise upon the foolish.

Sir William Osler
(1849-1919; Canadian physician)

✦ The physician's highest calling, his only calling, is to make sick people healthy — to heal, as it is termed.

Samuel Hahnemann
(1755-1843; German physician)

✦ Observation, reason, human understanding, courage; these make the physician.

Martin H. Fischer
(1879-1962; German-American physician & author)

✦ I think human beings have an innate desire to help each other. And whether you're in medicine or anything else, if you see someone that you can help... you get a gratification from doing it. In fact, I think that is perhaps the most important, you might say, fabric that holds the society together.

Michael E. DeBakey
(1908-2008; American cardiovascular surgeon)

✦ All labor that uplifts humanity has dignity and importance and should be undertaken with painstaking excellence.

Martin Luther King, Jr.
(1929-1968; American Baptist minister
& civil rights leader)

_____

✦ A wise physician, skill'd our wounds to heal, is more than armies to the public weal.

Alexander Pope
(1688-1744; English poet)

_____

✦ A well-trained, sensible doctor is one of the most valuable assets of a community.

Sir William Osler
(1849-1919; Canadian physician)

_____

✦ Trials are medicines which our gracious and wise
  physician prescribes because we need them; and he
  proportions the frequency and weight of them to what
  the case requires. Let us trust his skill and thank him for
  his prescription.

Sir Isaac Newton
(1643-1727; English mathematician,
physicist, astronomer, theologian, & author)

✦ Doctors and clergymen. A physician's physiology has
  much the same relation to his power of healing as a
  cleric's divinity has to his power of influencing conduct.

Samuel Butler
(1835-1902; English novelist)

✦ Men who are occupied in the restoration of health to
other men, by the joint exertion of skill and humanity, are
above all the great of the earth. They even partake of
divinity, since to preserve and renew is almost as noble
as to create.

Francois-Marie Arouet, known
by his nom de plume, Voltaire
(1694-1778; French writer & philosopher)

Chapter 2

A discipline where art, science, & philosophy merge

The best physician is also a philosopher.

Galen

(129 AD-210 AD; Greek physician & philosopher)

The practice of medicine and surgery, from its earliest beginnings to present day, remains a beautiful confluence of art, science, and philosophy. Whether or not we actively think about this concept, there is a constant balance and delicate interplay being employed to coalesce these three factors into a sound formula for success in providing safe and compassionate medical care for our ailing patients.

Medicine and surgery is the art of comforting and healing the mind, body, and soul through empathetic application of knowledge attained and experience acquired; the sound and meticulous employment of technical dexterities learned and practiced; strategically harnessing scientific principles with fastidious observation, reasoning, and methods; and partaking in regular philosophic thought to guide the path of healing forward.

As we pursue a commanding mastery of these disciplines throughout the course of our professional practice, let us strive to unite these fundamental factors of art, science, and philosophy in a manner which enables us to most effectively treat patients who are seeking care in our office, hospital, and operating theater.

DM

The physician should look upon the patient as a besieged city and try to rescue him with every means that art and science place at his command.
Alexander of Tralles
(525 AD-605 AD; Greek physician)

✦ We profess to teach the principles and practice of medicine, or, in other words, the science and art of medicine. Science is knowledge reduced to principles; art is knowledge reduced to practice. The knowing and doing, however, are distinct. ...Your knowledge, therefore, is useless unless you cultivate the art of healing. Unfortunately, the scientific man very often has the least amount of art, and he is totally unsuccessful in practice; and, on the other hand, there may be much art based on an infinitesimal amount of knowledge, and yet it is sufficient to make its cultivator eminent.

Sir Samuel Wilks
(1824-1911; British physician)

─────────────────────

✦ Every science touches art at some points — every art has its scientific side; the worst man of science is he who is never an artist, and the worst artist is he who is never a man of science.

Armand Trousseau
(1801-1867; French physician)

─────────────────────

✦ The art of science is as important as so-called technical science. You need both. It's this combination that must be recognized and acknowledged and valued.

Jonas Salk
(1914-1995; American medical researcher & virologist)

_____

✦ The great experimental principle, then, is doubt, that philosophic doubt which leaves to the mind its freedom and initiative, and from which the virtues most valuable to investigators in physiology and medicine are derived.

Claude Bernard
(1813-1878; French physiologist)

_____

✦ Medicine is a science of uncertainty and an art of probability.

Sir William Osler
(1849-1919; Canadian physician)

_____

✦ The forms of diseases are many and the healing of them is manifold.

Hippocrates
(460 BC-370 BC; Greek physician)

_____

✦ Medicine is a science, acquiring a practice an art.

Anonymous

_____

✦ As art is a habit with reference to things to be done, so is science a habit in respect to things to be known.

William Harvey
(1578-1657; English physician)

_____

✦ The philosophies of one age have become the absurdities of the next, and the foolishness of yesterday has become the wisdom of tomorrow.

Sir William Osler
(1849-1919; Canadian physician)

_____

✦ Medicine is the science by which we learn the various states of the human body in health and when not in health, and the means by which health is likely to be lost and, when lost, is likely to be restored back to health. In other words, it is the art whereby health is conserved and the art whereby it is restored after being lost. While some divide medicine into a theoretical and a practical science, others may assume that it is only theoretical because they see it as a pure science. But, in truth, every science has both a theoretical and a practical side.

Avicenna
(980 AD-1037 AD; Persian physician)

✦ Medicine is not only a science; it is also an art. It does not consist of compounding pills and plasters; it deals with the very processes of life, which must be understood before they may be guided.

Paracelsus
(1493-1541; Swiss physician)

✦ The dedicated physician is constantly striving from a balance between personal, human values, scientific realities and the inevitabilities of God's will.

David B. Allman
(1891-1971; American physician)

✦ Doctor Johnson said, that in sickness there were three things that were material; the physician, the disease, and the patient: and if any two of these joined, then they get the victory; for, *Ne Hercules quidem contra duos* [Not even Hercules himself is a match for two]. If the physician and the patient join, then down goes the disease; for then the patient recovers: if the physician and the disease join, that is a strong disease; and the physician mistaking the cure, then down goes the patient: if the patient and the disease join, then down goes the physician; for he is discredited.

Sir Francis Bacon
(1561-1626; English philosopher & statesman)

19

✦ The ordinary patient goes to his doctor because he is in pain or some other discomfort and wants to be comfortable again; he is not in pursuit of the ideal of health in any direct sense. The doctor on the other hand wants to discover the pathological condition and control it if he can. The two are thus to some degree at cross purposes from the first, and unless the affair is brought to an early and happy conclusion this diversion of aims is likely to become more and more serious as the case goes on.

Wilfred Trotter
(1872-1939; English surgeon)

✦ When the disease is stronger than the patient, the physician will not be able to help him at all, and if the strength of the patient is greater than the strength of the disease, he does not need a physician at all. But when both are equal, he needs a physician who will support the patient's strength and help him against the disease.

Rhazes
(854 AD-925 AD; Persian physician & philosopher)

✦ Medicine deals with the states of health and disease in the human body. It is a truism of philosophy that a complete knowledge of a thing can only be obtained by elucidating its causes and antecedents, provided, of course, such causes exist. In medicine it is, therefore, necessary that causes of both health and disease should be determined.

Avicenna
(980 AD-1037 AD; Persian physician)

✦ The theory of medicine, therefore, presents what is useful in thought, but does not indicate how it is to be applied in practice — the mode of operation of these principles. The theory, when mastered, gives us a certain kind of knowledge. Thus we say, for example, there are three forms of fevers and nine constitutions. The practice of medicine is not the work which the physician carries out, but is that branch of medical knowledge which, when acquired, enables one to form an opinion upon which to base the proper plan of treatment.

Avicenna
(980 AD-1037 AD; Persian physician)

Chapter 3

First do no harm — primum non nocere

The physician must be able to tell the antecedents, know the present, and foretell the future — must mediate these things, and have two special objects in view with regard to disease, namely, to do good or to do no harm.

Hippocrates
(460 BC-370 BC; Greek physician)

● *We should all recall this fundamental precept of the Hippocratic Oath and strive to preserve its ancient but ceaseless and vital guidance in the forefront of our clinical minds. "First do no harm."*

Never act in vain if a particular treatment, esoteric test, imaging study, or procedure will not serve to truly change your management and may only further the complexity of any given clinical situation to no avail. In fact, these unwarranted interventions may only serve to propagate an ineffectual cycle of unnecessary diagnostic testing and invasive procedures that ultimately will not add to the good of the patient. Furthermore, this path may subject the patient to pain and suffering that is of little or no benefit.

In executing the art of medicine, we must remember to ask ourselves, "Will this change my management?" and, "Will the benefits of the proposed clinical course of action outweigh the potential risks?" Be mindful of taking for granted the seemingly unlimited ability, at most modern medical institutions, to order and obtain any and every diagnostic test or imaging study imaginable.

Take note of the following Chinese proverb which wisely states, "The patient has two sleeves, one containing a diagnostic and the other a therapeutic armamentarium; these sleeves should rarely be emptied in one move; keep some techniques in reserve; time your maneuvers to best serve the status and special needs of your patient."

If actionable diagnostic intelligence is obtained or impactful results are achieved through diagnostic studies or invasive procedures performed, respectively, then by all means pursue this course of action when warranted. However, if these diagnostic and therapeutic arrows will be of limited utility, serve only to cloud the clinical picture, or subject your patient to pain, discomfort, and mental anguish, they must remain safely stowed in a quiver rather than being flung haphazardly down-range at a nebulous target.

I tell my patients who are undergoing common operations or procedures, no matter how small the procedure may be, that there is no such thing as a "routine" or "minor" procedure. Ultimately, we have no absolute prophetic mechanism to predict when a complication may occur, how serious it may be, and how much of a toll it will ultimately take upon the patient. No operation or procedure is absolutely "routine" or "minor" and we should not take this description for granted when discussing operations and procedures with our patients.

We should ultimately aim to heal and to alleviate pain, pathology, and suffering; however, our primary quest as healers should first and foremost be to not do harm.

DM

In the performance of our duty one feeling should direct us;
the case we should consider as our own, and we should ask
ourselves, whether, placed under similar circumstances, we
should choose to submit to the pain and danger we are about
to inflict.

Sir Astley Paston Cooper
(1768-1841; English surgeon & anatomist)

✦ Only one rule in medical ethics need concern you — that action on your part which best conserves the interest of your patient.

Martin H. Fischer
(1879-1962; German-American physician & author)

✦ Into whatsoever houses I enter, I will enter to help the sick, and I will abstain from all intentional wrong-doing and harm, especially from abusing the bodies of man or woman, bond or free. And whatsoever I shall see or hear in the course of my profession, as well as outside my profession in my intercourse with men, if it be what should not be published abroad, I will never divulge, holding such things to be holy secrets.

Hippocrates
(460 BC-370 BC; Greek physician)

✦ I trust I may be enabled in the treatment of patients always to act with a single eye to their good.

Joseph Lister
(1827-1912; British surgeon & physician)

✦ The highest ideal of cure is the speedy, gentle, and enduring restoration of health by the most trustworthy and least harmful way.

Samuel Hahnemann
(1755-1843; German physician)

✦ Whenever a doctor cannot do good, he must be kept from doing harm.

Hippocrates
(460 BC-370 BC; Greek physician)

✦ I never say of an operation that it is without danger.

August Bier
(1861-1949; German surgeon)

✦ Make a habit of two things: to help; or at least to do no harm.

Hippocrates
(460 BC-370 BC; Greek physician)

✦ The physician, to the extent he is a physician, considers
   only the good of the patient in what he prescribes, and
   his own not at all.

Plato
(~428 BC–~347 BC; Greek philosopher)

✦ It is no part of a physician's business to use either
   persuasion or compulsion upon the patients.

Aristotle
(384 BC–322 BC; Greek philosopher)

✦ Surgeons must be very careful
   When they take the knife!
   Underneath their fine incisions
   Stirs the Culprit – Life!

Emily Dickinson
(1830–1886; American poet)

Chapter 4

The history & physical examination: every patient has a story to tell

Listen to your patient, he is telling you the diagnosis.

Sir William Osler

(1849-1919; Canadian physician)

Taking a thorough clinical history and performing a proper physical examination comprise the bedrock of a patient-physician relationship. This relationship must be tenderly cultivated as a means to building rapport with patients as well as to facilitate a sound approach to the implementation of diagnostic and therapeutic interventions.

This clinical responsibility in some circumstances seems to have become a lost art. In the modern era of medicine, with increasingly time-constrained patient encounters, there is a tendency to rapidly collect a chief complaint followed shortly thereafter by launching an impressive salvo of diagnostic tests rather than taking an appropriate history and performing a thorough physical examination. While the temptation may be present, we should never allow laboratory tests nor imaging studies to serve as a substitute for the irreplaceable value of a thorough clinical history and physical examination.

In addition to an educated clinical mind, the most valuable clinical dexterities a physician can hone as a means to delivering excellent patient care are our eyes, ears, and hands. Neither a CT scan, MRI, nor complex panel of laboratory studies could ever replace the value of a well-executed history and physical examination. Before gathering objective laboratory and radiographic data let your senses guide your observations, reasoning, and methods. Eighty percent, or more, of clinical diagnoses can be arrived upon by a thorough history and physical examination alone.

It is of utmost importance that we continually strive to cultivate and sharpen our clinical skill, prowess, and acumen *with the five senses that have been innately provided to us. Moreover, we must ensure this crucial skill set is aptly taught to the future generations of healthcare professionals learning and growing under our tutelage. If this critical skill set is lost we will have squandered the very foundation of which the art of medicine and surgery has been built upon.*

DM

When you no longer know what headache, heartache, or stomachache means without cistern punctures, electrocardiograms and six X-ray plates, you are slipping.

Martin H. Fischer

(1879-1962; German-American physician & author)

✦ Every physician must be rich in knowledge, and not only of that which is written in books; his patients should be his book, they will never mislead him.

Paracelsus
(1493-1541; Swiss physician)

✦ Let the young know they will never find a more interesting, more instructive book than the patient himself.

Giorgio Baglivi
(1668-1707; Italian physician)

✦ The doctor may also learn more about the illness from the way the patient tells the story than from the story itself.

James B. Herrick
(1861-1954; American physician)

✦ In acute diseases the physician must conduct his inquiries in the following way. First he must examine the face of the patient, and see whether it is like the faces of healthy people, and especially whether it is like its usual self. Such likeness will be the best sign, and the greatest unlikeness will be the most dangerous sign. The latter will be as follows. Nose sharp, eyes hollow, temples sunken, ears cold and contracted with their lobes turned outwards, the skin about the face hard and tense and parched, the colour of the face as a whole being yellow or black.

Hippocrates
(460 BC-370 BC; Greek physician)

_____

✦ Learn to listen with your fingers.

Helen Taussig
(1898-1986; American cardiologist)

_____

✦ Observe, record, tabulate, communicate. Use your five senses. Learn to see, learn to hear, learn to feel, learn to smell, and know that by practice alone you can become expert.

Sir William Osler
(1849-1919; Canadian physician)

✦ Where a man feels pain he lays his hand.

Dutch proverb

✦ The first [quality] to be named must always be the power of attention, of giving one's whole mind to the patient without the interposition of oneself. It sounds simple but only the very greatest doctors ever fully attain it...

Wilfred Trotter
(1872-1939; English surgeon)

✦ Symptoms, then, are in reality nothing but a cry from suffering organs.

Jean-Martin Charcot
(1825- 1893; French neurologist)

✦ If migraine patients have a common and legitimate second complaint besides their migraines, it is that they have not been listened to by physicians. Looked at, investigated, drugged, charged, but not listened to.

Oliver Sacks
(1933-2015; British neurologist & author)

✦ The two fulcra of medicine are reason and observation. Observation is the clue to guide the physician in his thinking.

Giorgio Baglivi
(1668-1707; Italian physician)

✦   The student is to collect and evaluate facts. The facts are locked up in the patient.

Abraham Flexner
(1866-1959; American educator)

―――――――――――――――――――

✦   There is only one cardinal rule: one must always listen to the patient.

Oliver Sacks
(1933-2015; British neurologist & author)

―――――――――――――――――――

Chapter 5

Battle disease with your head & heart in equal measure: empathy, compassion, reassurance, & bedside manner

Medicine is not merely a science but an art. The character of the physician may act more powerfully upon the patient than the drugs employed.

Paracelsus
(1493-1541; Swiss physician)

● *The merits of empathy, compassion, and reassurance, which directly contribute to a physician's "bedside manner," are without a doubt among the most valuable tools a physician may draw from in his or her armamentarium when preparing* for battle against illness and injury. It is these virtues that may very well prove to be the sharpest therapeutic instruments or the most potent of potions you possess in your black leather physician's bag.

The importance of this concept is overwhelmingly evident in the large body of historic medical literature and was clearly recognized as an invaluable tool by physicians throughout history as illustrated in the following quotes. These values are as old as the discipline of medicine itself although they steadfastly remain key pillars of humanistic medical care, as they always will.

The 19th century American sociologist, Lewis G. Janes, once wrote, "Disease is war with the laws of our being, and all war, as a great general has said, is hell." Thus, heed the empathetic advice offered by Plato himself, "Be kind. Every person you meet is fighting a difficult battle."

The head and the heart must be actively engaged, employed, and exercised against malady and affliction in equal measure as we execute our healing art. When these powers are brought to bear against the pathologic forces of disease, you and your patient will undoubtedly possess a strategic advantage for victory.

DM

Sufficient knowledge and a solid background in the basic sciences are essential for all medical students. But that is not enough. A physician is not only a scientist or a good technician. He must be more than that — he must have good human qualities. He has to have a personal understanding and sympathy for the suffering of human beings.

Albert Einstein
(1879-1955; German physicist)

✦ The art of medicine has its roots in the heart.

Paracelsus
(1493-1541; Swiss physician)

_____

✦ Wherever the art of medicine is loved, there is also a love of humanity.

Hippocrates
(460 BC-370 BC; Greek physician)

_____

✦ The highest degree of a medicine is Love.

Paracelsus
(1493-1541; Swiss physician)

_____

✦ Kindness which is bestowed on the good is never lost.

Plato
(~428 BC-~347 BC; Greek philosopher)

_____

✦ Cure sometimes, treat often, comfort always.

Hippocrates
(460 BC-370 BC; Greek physician)

✦ Care more for the individual patient than for the special features of the disease... Put yourself in his place... The kindly word, the cheerful greeting, the sympathetic look — these the patient understands.

Sir William Osler
(1849-1919; Canadian physician)

✦ It is not a case we are treating; it is a living, palpitating, alas, too often suffering fellow creature.

John Brown
(1810-1882; Scottish physician)

✦ The dedicated doctor knows that he must be both scientist and humanitarian; his most agonizing decisions lie in the field of human relations.

David B. Allman
(1891-1971; American physician)

✦ There is a wisdom of the head, and... a wisdom of the heart.

Charles Dickens
(1812-1870; English novelist)

✦ Educating the mind without educating the heart is no education at all.

Aristotle
(384 BC-322 BC; Greek philosopher)

✦ Often the confidence of the patient in his physician does more for the cure of his disease than the physician with all his remedies.

Henri de Mondeville
(1260-1320; French surgeon)

✦ In the sick room, ten cents' worth of human understanding equals ten dollars' worth of medical science.

Martin H. Fischer
(1879-1962; German-American physician & author)

✦ For some patients, though conscious that their condition is perilous, recover their health simply through their contentment with the goodness of the physician.

Hippocrates
(460 BC-370 BC; Greek physician)

✦ Courtesy is as much a mark of a gentleman as courage.

Theodore Roosevelt
(1858-1919; American statesman, politician, conservationist,
naturalist, writer & 26th President of the United States)

✦ Each patient ought to feel somewhat the better after the physician's visit, irrespective of the nature of the illness.

Warfield Theobald Longcope
(1877-1953; American physician)

✦ The physician must not only be the healer, but often the consoler.

Harriot Kezia Hunt
(1805-1875; American physician)

✦ Let your entrance into the sick room decrease, not increase, the irritability of your patient.

Martin H. Fischer
(1879-1962; German-American physician & author)

✦ To array a man's will against his sickness is the supreme art of medicine.

Henry Ward Beecher
(1813-1887; American clergyman)

✦ A little flattery will support a man through great fatigue.

James Monroe
(1758-1831; 5th President of the United States)

✦ Drugs are not always necessary. Belief in recovery always
   is.

> **Norman Cousins**
> **(1915-1990; American journalist & author)**

✦ Hope awakens courage. He who can implant courage in
   the human soul is the best physician.

> **Karl Ludwig von Knebel**
> **(1744-1834; German poet)**

✦ He is the best physician who is the most ingenious
   inspirer of hope.

> **Samuel Taylor Coleridge**
> **(1772-1834; English poet & philosopher)**

✦ You must learn to talk clearly. The jargon of scientific
   terminology which rolls off your tongues is mental
   garbage.

> **Martin H. Fischer**
> **(1879-1962; German-American physician & author)**

✦ Before you tell the 'truth' to the patient, be sure you
   know the 'truth' and that the patient wants to hear it.
   Chinese proverb

   _____

✦ The patient does not care about your science; what he
   wants to know is, can you cure him?
   Martin H. Fischer
   (1879-1962; German-American physician & author)

   _____

✦ If your news must be bad, tell it soberly and promptly.
   Henry Howarth Bashford
   (1880-1961; English physician & author)

   _____

✦ Medicine would be the ideal profession if it did not
   involve giving pain.
   Samuel Hopkins Adams
   (1871-1958; American writer)

   _____

✦ A physician is not angry at the intemperance of a mad patient, nor does he take it ill to be railed at by a man in fever. Just so should a wise man treat all mankind, as a physician does his patient, and look upon them only as sick and extravagant.

Seneca
(4 BC-65 AD; Roman philosopher & statesman)

✦ It is the surgeon's duty to tranquilize the temper, to beget cheerfulness, and to impart confidence of recovery.

Sir Astley Paston Cooper
(1768-1841; English surgeon & anatomist)

✦ Let the surgeon take care to regulate the whole regimen of the patient's life for joy and happiness by promising that he will soon be well, by allowing his relatives and special friends to cheer him and by having someone tell him jokes, and let him be solaced also by music on the viol or psaltery. The surgeon must forbid anger, hatred, and sadness in the patient, and remind him that the body grows fat from joy and thin from sadness.

Henri de Mondeville
(1260-1320; French surgeon)

✦ When a doctor arrives to attend some patient of the working class, he ought not to feel his pulse the moment he enters, as is nearly always done without regard to the circumstances of the man who lies sick; he should not remain standing while he considers what he ought to do, as though the fate of a human being were a mere trifle; rather let him condescend to sit down for awhile.

Bernardino Ramazzini
(1633-1714; Italian physician)

✦ They may forget your name, but they will never forget how you made them feel.

Carl W. Buehner
(1898-1974; General authority of
The Church of Jesus Christ of Latter-day Saints)

✦ It is not how much you do, but how much love you put into the doing that matters.

Mother Teresa
(1910-1997; Roman Catholic nun & missionary)

✦ People pay the doctor for his trouble; for his kindness they still remain in his debt.

Seneca
(4 BC-65 AD; Roman philosopher & statesman)

Chapter 6

Heal the whole patient: see the forest, not the trees

The cure of the part should not be attempted without treatment of the whole. No attempt should be made to cure the body without the soul. Let no one persuade you to cure the head until he has first given you his soul to be cured, for this is the great error of our day, that physicians first separate the soul from the body.

Plato
(~428 BC-~347 BC; Greek philosopher)

● *Our patients are not wickets, they are not widgets, and they should not be measured as productivity units. They are* living, breathing, and suffering from malady and affliction. Treat the patient sitting in your office or lying on the hospital gurney, not the digitized high-resolution computer-generated imaging studies or slew of laboratory results. Concomitantly treat the mind, body, and soul of your patients with all the respect each of these parts deserve and this strategy will never lead you astray. When you treat each of these variables in concert, the result of treating the patient as a whole becomes synergistic, and the sum of your efforts will be greater than the equal value of the parts.

Each patient possesses unique social circumstances. Each patient harbors a unique physical, psychological, and physiologic composition. Furthermore, patients and the presentation of illnesses do not always adhere to the objective medical and scientific parameters held within the pages of the hallowed medical texts we are reared upon.

Claude Bernard, a 19th century French physiologist suggested, "Effects vary with the conditions which bring them to pass, but laws do not vary. Physiological and pathological states are ruled by the same forces; they differ only because of the special conditions under which the vital laws manifest themselves."

In some way or another each case we treat is unique. Each case requires cognizant management of the mind, body, and soul to ultimately facilitate healing.

DM

Variability is the law of life, and as no two faces are the same, so no two bodies are alike, and no two individuals react alike and behave alike under the abnormal conditions which we know as disease.

Sir William Osler
(1849-1919; Canadian physician)

✦   Anyone who believes that anything can be suited to
    everyone is a great fool, because medicine is practised not
    on mankind in general, but on every individual in
    particular.

Henri de Mondeville
(1260-1320; French surgeon)

✦   It is more important to know what sort of person has a
    disease than to know what sort of disease a person has.

Hippocrates
(460 BC-370 BC; Greek physician)

✦   If it were not for the great variability among individuals,
    medicine might as well be a science, not an art.

Sir William Osler
(1849-1919; Canadian physician)

✦ A physician is obligated to consider more than a diseased organ, more even than the whole man — he must view the man in his world.

Harvey Cushing
(1869-1939; American neurosurgeon & writer)

✦ The physician must give heed to the region in which the patient lives, that is to say, to its type and peculiarities.

Paracelsus
(1493-1541; Swiss physician)

✦ A careful physician... before he attempts to administer a remedy to his patient, must investigate not only the malady of the man he wishes to cure, but also his habits when in health, and his physical constitution.

Marcus Tullius Cicero
(106 BC-43 BC; Roman statesman & philosopher)

✦ The good physician treats the disease; the great physician treats the patient who has the disease.

Sir William Osler

(1849-1919; Canadian physician)

✦ The cure of many diseases remains unknown to the physicians of Hellos (Greece) because they do not study the whole person.

Socrates

(470 BC-399 BC; Greek philosopher)

✦ The physician should not treat the disease but the patient who is suffering from it.

Maimonides

(~1135 AD-1204 AD; Jewish physician & philosopher)

✦ Life is short, and the Art long; the occasion fleeting; experience fallacious, and judgment difficult. The physician must not only be prepared to do what is right himself, but also to make the patient, the attendants, and externals cooperate.

Hippocrates
(460 BC-370 BC; Greek physician)

✦ Body and soul cannot be separated for purposes of treatment, for they are one and indivisible. Sick minds must be healed as well as sick bodies.

Jeff C. Miller
(1874-1936; American physician)

✦ The greatest mistake in the treatment of diseases is that there are physicians for the body and physicians for the soul, although the two cannot be separated.

Plato
(~428 BC-~347 BC; Greek philosopher)

✦ The mind, in addition to medicine, has powers to turn the immune system around.

Jonas Salk
(1914-1995; American medical researcher & virologist)

_____

✦ When you treat a disease, first treat the mind.

Chen Jen

_____

✦ Never forget that it is not a pneumonia, but a pneumonic man who is your patient.

Sir William Withey Gull
(1816-1890; English physician)

_____

✦ Treat the patient, not the X-ray.

James M. Hunter
(1924-2013; American surgeon)

_____

✦ In examining disease, we gain wisdom about anatomy
and physiology and biology. In examining the person
with disease, we gain wisdom about life.

Oliver Sacks
(1933-2015; British neurologist & author)

✦ The cure of many diseases is unknown to physicians
because they are ignorant of the whole... For the part can
never be well unless the whole is well.

Plato
(~428 BC-~347 BC; Greek philosopher)

Chapter 7

The unrelenting shadow of the scythe

Tis not always in a physician's power to cure the sick; at
times the disease is stronger than trained art.

Ovid
(43 BC-~18 AD; Roman poet)

● *Despite our best and most genuine efforts, as well as
employment of the powerful and vast advances we have
harnessed in modern medicine, at times there are
unconquerable forces of disease at play that we as physicians
cannot surmount. When a terminally ill patient, or a patient we*

no longer have the capability to save, passes from the living world at their time of death, this should not be seen as defeat. It should be seen as mercy from suffering that the offending pathology has produced. This we must accept as an unfortunate but inevitable truth of our profession. We must resolve to keep moving forward. We must continue carrying out the healing art and science of medicine and surgery to the best of our ability so that we may help as many others as possible.

DM

A physician can sometimes parry the scythe of death, but has no power over the sand in the hourglass.

Hester Lynch Piozzi
(1741-1821; English author)

✦ There is only one ultimate and effectual preventative for the maladies to which flesh is heir, and that is death.

Harvey Cushing
(1869-1939; American neurosurgeon & writer)

✦ When he can render no further aid, the physician alone can mourn as a man with his incurable patient. This is the physician's sad lot.

Aretaeus of Cappadocia
(1st century AD; Greek physician)

✦ The prime goal is to alleviate suffering, and not to prolong life. And if your treatment does not alleviate suffering, but only prolongs life, that treatment should be stopped.

Christiaan Barnard
(1922-2001; South African cardiac surgeon)

✦ If the just cure of a disease be full of peril, let the
physician resort to palliation.

Sir Francis Bacon
(1561-1626; English philosopher & statesman)

✦ I believe often that death is good medical treatment
because it can achieve what all the medical advances and
technology cannot achieve today, and that is stop the
suffering of the patient.

Christiaan Barnard
(1922-2001; South African cardiac surgeon)

✦ The rich man, gasping for breath... feels at last the
impotence of gold; that death which he dreaded at a
distance as an enemy, he now hails when he is near, as a
friend; a friend that alone can bring the peace his
treasures cannot purchase, and remove the pain his
physicians cannot cure.

Charles Caleb Colton
(1780-1832; English writer)

✦ Everything but truth becomes loathed in a sick-room.
...Let the nurse avow that the medicine is nauseous. Let
the physician declare that the treatment will be painful.
Let sister, or brother, or friend, tell me that I must never
look to be well. When the time approaches that I am to
die, let me be told that I am to die, and when.

Harriet Martineau
(1802-1876; British writer & sociologist)

✦ By medicine life may be prolong'd, yet death
Will seize the doctor too.

William Shakespeare
(1564-1616; English poet & playwright)

Part II

PILLARS OF TIMELESS WISDOM FOR CLINICAL PRACTICE

The universities do not teach all things... so a doctor
must seek out old wives, gypsies, sorcerers, wandering
tribes, old robbers, and such outlaws and take lessons
from them. A doctor must be a traveller... Knowledge is
experience.

Paracelsus
(1493-1541; Swiss physician)

Chapter 8

Medical education, training, & learning

Medicine is learned by the bedside and not in the classroom. Let not your conceptions of disease come from words heard in the lecture room or read from the book. See, and then reason and compare and control. But see first.

Sir William Osler

(1849-1919; Canadian physician)

● As medical professionals we should always remain faithful and humble students. We should always continue honing our craft through a lifetime of professional learning.

Being a perpetually dutiful student, committed to life-long learning, is the only way to keep pace with the ever expanding field of medicine as it continues to boldly forge ahead.

The value of real hands-on clinical learning by accosting the examination table in outpatient offices, the bedside on the clinical wards, and the operating table in the operating theaters will eternally remain the ultimate classroom for medical education. This is eloquently described in the quotes to follow which have been conferred upon us by the likes of Sir William Osler, the infamous "father of modern medicine" and architect of the contemporary structure of postgraduate medical education, among others.

There simply is no substitute for real hands-on clinical learning. Simulation-based education has taken root as an effort to enhance this aspect of medial training, and is important in its own right; however, there is no substitute for learning through real life patient care. Nor will there ever be. To learn the true art and craft of medicine, students must dutifully patrol the wards, they must learn their way around the laboratory and radiographic suites, they must partake in the activities of the operating theaters, and most importantly of all, they must see the bedsheets and what lies beneath!

DM

He who studies medicine without books sails an uncharted sea, but he who studies medicine without patients does not go to sea at all.

Sir William Osler
(1849-1919; Canadian physician)

✦ To have a group of cloistered clinicians away completely from the broad current of professional life would be bad for teacher and worse for student. The primary work of a professor of medicine in a medical school is in the wards, teaching his pupils how to deal with patients and their diseases.

Sir William Osler
(1849-1919; Canadian physician)

✦ There are two objects of medical education: to heal the sick and to advance the science.

Charles H. Mayo
(1865-1939; American physician)

✦ Learning is the only thing the mind never exhausts, never fears, and never regrets.

Leonardo da Vinci
(1452-1519; Italian Renaissance man)

✦ It is what we know already that often prevents us from learning.

Claude Bernard
(1813-1878; French physiologist)

_____

✦ Education is not learning, but the training of the mind that it may learn.

Sir William Withey Gull
(1816-1890; English physician)

_____

✦ Man can learn nothing unless he proceeds from the known to the unknown.

Claude Bernard
(1813-1878; French physiologist)

_____

✦ The higher education so much needed today is not given in the school, is not to be bought in the market place, but it has to be wrought out in each one of us for himself; it is the silent influence of character on character.

Sir William Osler
(1849-1919; Canadian physician)

_____

75

✦ Education comes from within; you get it by struggle and effort and thought.

Napoleon Hill
(1883-1970; American author)

✦ Medical education is not just a program for building knowledge and skills in its recipients... it is also an experience which creates attitudes and expectations.

Abraham Flexner
(1866-1959; American educator)

✦ This is all very fine, but it won't do — Anatomy — Botany — Nonsense! Sir, I know an old woman in Covent Garden, who understands botany better, and as for anatomy, my butcher can dissect a joint full as well; no, young man, all that is stuff; you must go to the bedside, it is there alone you can learn disease!

Thomas Sydenham
(1624-1689; English physician)

✦ The road to medical knowledge is through the pathological museum and not through an apothecary's shop.

> **Sir William Withey Gull**
> **(1816-1890; English physician)**

✦ The doors of wisdom are never shut.

> **Benjamin Franklin**
> **(1706-1790; author, inventor,**
> **scientist, politician, & statesman)**

✦ I profess to learn and to teach anatomy not from books but from dissections, not from the tenets of philosophers but from the fabric of nature.

> **William Harvey**
> **(1578-1657; English physician)**

✦ Every patient you see is a lesson in much more than the malady from which he suffers. The hardest conviction to get into the mind of a beginner is that the education upon which he is engaged is not a college course, not a medical course, but a life course, for which the work of a few years under teachers is but a preparation.

Sir William Osler
(1849-1919; Canadian physician)

✦ The student of medicine can no more hope to advance in the mastery of his subject with a loose and careless mind than the student of mathematics. If the laws of abstract truth require such rigid precision from those who study them, we cannot believe the laws of nature require less. On the contrary, they would seem to require more; for the facts are obscure, the means of inquiry imperfect, and in every exercise of the mind there are peculiar facilities to err.

Sir William Withey Gull
(1816-1890; English physician)

✦ Too many men slip early out of the habit of studious reading, and yet that is essential.

Sir William Osler
(1849-1919; Canadian physician)

✦ Real education must ultimately be limited to men who insist on knowing, the rest is mere sheep-herding.

Ezra Pound
(1885-1972; American poet)

✦ To become comfortable with uncertainty is one of the primary goals in the training of a physician.

Sherwin B. Nuland
(1930-2014; American surgeon & writer)

✦ What is education? Teaching a man what his powers and relations are, and how he can best extend, strengthen, and employ them.

Sir William Withey Gull
(1816-1890; English physician)

79

✦ A good teacher must know the rules; a good pupil, the exceptions.

Martin H. Fischer
(1879-1962; German-American physician & author)

✦ War is the only proper school of the surgeon.

Hippocrates
(460 BC-370 BC; Greek physician)

✦ The better educated we are and the more acquired information we have, the better prepared shall we find our minds for making great and fruitful discoveries.

Claude Bernard
(1813-1878; French physiologist)

✦ Medicine is essentially a learned profession. Its literature is ancient, and connects it with the most learned periods of antiquity; and its terminology continues to be Greek or Latin. You cannot name a part of the body, and scarcely a disease, without the use of a classical term. Every structure bears upon it the impress of learning, and is a silent appeal to the student to cultivate an acquaintance with the sources from which the nomenclature of his profession is derived.

Sir William Withey Gull
(1816-1890; English physician)

✦   What is the student but a lover courting a fickle mistress who ever eludes his grasp?

Sir William Osler
(1849-1919; Canadian physician)

Chapter 9

Experience: the ultimate clinical compass

The art of medicine was to be properly learned only from its practice and its exercise.

Thomas Sydenham
(1624-1689; English physician)

● *The most potent, unforgiving, and righteous teacher we can receive tutelage from as we pursue excellence in the practice of medicine is that of experience. In the same vein, at certain times the most valuable clinical ally you will possess and can rely upon is that of your own prior clinical experience.*

The legendary Leonardo da Vinci asserted the opinion that, "Experience is a truer guide than the words of others." This sentiment is certainly applicable to the practice of medicine as it is in the larger context of life. The 15th century Swiss physician, Paracelsus, wisely parallels this perspective as it relates to the practice of medicine by expressing, "The art of medicine cannot be inherited, nor can it be copied from books."

Lessons learned, for better or for worse, as we proceed through the peaks and valleys of our careers are seared into the fiber and psyche of our being. These experiences can be an incredibly powerful influence. They harbor the capacity to prudently affect our clinical decision-making processes and can wisely guide us in a way that could never be attained from books nor didactic lectures.

We will all inevitably encounter difficult cases, complications, and clinical complexities. Embrace and utilize the powerful tool of experience when the way ahead seems uncertain and perilous. When searching in vain for a path forward through these clinical challenges, when it seems an impasse has been encountered and the clinical true north cannot be reckoned, consult the compass of clinical experience to guide the way.

In addition to learning from one's own experiences, we should also capitalize on absorbing the lessons of experience from those mentors, senior clinicians, and historic giants of medicine and surgery who have come before us. They have walked in our shoes and they have trodden the same clinical paths we find ourselves warily travelling. The breadth of knowledge available which can be derived from the experiences of others is astounding. Therefore, let us resolve to acquire the wisdom embedded in the experience of our predecessors and implement these invaluable lessons learned. In doing so we may be able to circumvent our own missteps and failures as opposed to foolishly repeating them.

DM

It gives me great pleasure to converse with the aged. They have been over the road that all of us must travel, and know where it is rough and difficult and where it is level and easy.

Plato
(~428 BC-~347 BC; Greek philosopher)

✦ Even in populous districts, the practice of medicine is a lonely road which winds up-hill all the way and a man may easily go astray and never reach the Delectable Mountains unless he early finds those shepherd guides of whom Bunyan tells, Knowledge, Experience, Watchful, and Sincere.

Sir William Osler
(1849-1919; Canadian physician)

_____

✦ Observe the practice of many physicians; do not implicitly believe the mere assertion of your master; be something better than servile learner; go forth yourselves to see and compare!

Armand Trousseau
(1801-1867; French physician)

_____

✦ A wisdom deficit — fewer elders and even fewer people who listen to them.

Jonas Salk
(1914-1995; American medical researcher & virologist)

_____

✦ The value of experience is not in seeing much, but in seeing wisely.

Sir William Osler
(1849-1919; Canadian physician)

✦ I think of evolution as an error-making and error-correcting process, and we are constantly learning from experience.

Jonas Salk
(1914-1995; American medical researcher & virologist)

✦ There is no perfect knowledge which can be entitled ours, that is innate; none but what has been obtained from experience, or derived in some way from our senses.

William Harvey
(1578-1657; English physician)

✦ Experience is the great teacher; unfortunately, experience leaves mental scars, and scar tissue contracts.

William James Mayo
(1861-1939; American surgeon)

✦ We are constantly misled by the ease with which our minds fall into the ruts of one or two experiences.

Sir William Osler
(1849-1919; Canadian physician)

✦ Surgical knowledge depends on long practice, not from speculations.

Marcello Malpighi
(1628-1694; Italian physician & biologist)

✦ It is courage based on confidence, not daring, and it is confidence based on experience.

Jonas Salk
(1914-1995; American medical researcher & virologist)

✦ An event experienced is an event perceived, digested, and assimilated into the substance of our being, and the ratio between the number of cases seen and the number of cases assimilated is the measure of experience.

Wilfred Trotter
(1872-1939; English surgeon)

✦ The young physician starts life with 20 drugs for each disease, and the old physician ends life with one drug for 20 diseases.

Sir William Osler
(1849-1919; Canadian physician)

✦ Don't despise empiric truth. Lots of things work in practice for which the laboratory has never found proof.

Martin H. Fischer
(1879-1962; German-American physician & author)

✦ Nothing happens quite by chance. It's a question of accretion of information and experience.

Jonas Salk
(1914-1995; American medical researcher & virologist)

✦ Reasoning draws a conclusion, but does not make the conclusion certain, unless the mind discovers it by the path of experience.

Roger Bacon
(~1219-1292; English philosopher)

Chapter 10

Common sense: an uncommon virtue

Simplex sigillum veri: simplicity is the seal of truth.
Herman Boerhaave
(1668-1738; Dutch botanist, chemist, & physician)

● While human nature drives most of us to egotistically believe we possess boat loads of common sense as ballast to draw from in maintaining an even keel, let's be honest with ourselves; how often is common sense overlooked and underutilized? While zebras certainly lurk about our offices and hospital wards, common afflictions remain common, and common sense should remain the foundation for diagnosing and treating illness and injury.

Heed the advice of the 14th century English philosopher, Friar William of Ockham, who simply but elegantly coined the concept of "Ockham's razor." Novacula Occami — Ockham's razor, also known as lex parsimoniae (the law of parsimony), asserts that the simpler answer or solution for any given problem is most likely the correct course of action as opposed to a more complex answer or solution.

Always maintain a wary eye for zebras skirting the horizon of the savannahs in the African Serengeti. Nonetheless, primarily focus your efforts on common diagnoses and common cures. This approach, more often than not, will serve your patients with much greater potency than stalking exotic prey and pursuing uncommon diagnoses and complex interventions.

When in a clinical pinch, begin your problem-solving quest by exercising good plain common sense.

DM

The physician would be even worse off than he is, if not for the occasional emergence of common sense which breaks through dogmas with intuitive freshness.

Alexander Goldenweiser
(1880-1940; Russian-American anthropologist & sociologist)

✦ Common sense in matters medical is rare, and is usually in inverse ratio to the degree of education.

Sir William Osler
(1849-1919; Canadian physician)

✦ The best physician is he who can distinguish the possible from the impossible.

Herophilos
(335 BC-280 BC; Greek physician)

✦ The right question is usually more important than the right answer.

Plato
(~428 BC-~347 BC; Greek philosopher)

✦ This problem, once solved, will be simple.

Thomas Edison
(1847-1931; American inventor)

✦ Soap and water and common sense are the best disinfectants.

Sir William Osler
(1849-1919; Canadian physician)

✦ Common sense in an uncommon degree is what the world calls wisdom.

Samuel Taylor Coleridge
(1772-1834; English poet & philosopher)

✦ Truth is ever to be found in the simplicity, and not in the multiplicity and confusion of things.

Sir Isaac Newton
(1643-1727; English mathematician,
physicist, astronomer, theologian, & author)

✦ Common sense is something that everyone needs, few have, and none think they lack.

Benjamin Franklin
(1706-1790; author, inventor,
scientist, politician, & statesman)

✦ Knowledge is a process of piling up facts; wisdom lies in their simplification.

Martin H. Fischer
(1879-1962; German-American physician & author)

✦ Nature is pleased with simplicity. And nature is no dummy.

Sir Isaac Newton
(1643-1727; English mathematician,
physicist, astronomer, theologian, & author)

✦ Common sense without education, is better than education without common sense.

Benjamin Franklin
(1706-1790; author, inventor,
scientist, politician, & statesman)

✦ Simplicity is the ultimate sophistication.

Leonardo da Vinci
(1452-1519; Italian Renaissance man)

✦ Life is really simple, but we insist on making it complicated.

Confucius
(551 BC-479 BC; Chinese philosopher)

Chapter 11

The bitter taste of medicine

It is an art of no little importance to administer medicines properly: but, it is an art of much greater and more difficult acquisition to know when to suspend or altogether to omit them.

Philippe Pinel
(1745-1826; French physician)

● As physicians we have an unbelievably wide breadth of potions, pills, powders, poultices, lotions, ointments, creams, salves, tonics, inoculations, injections, and infusions readily *available and at our disposal to employ against the maladies that afflict our patients. While pharmacology is one of the most potent and important arms of modern medicine, let us not forget that these therapeutic regimens also possess deleterious effects and they are not always innocuous. It is these untoward effects that our patients will most vividly remember... In some cases these undesirable medicament effects must be endured to ultimately topple the pathologic adversary with which we battle. However, let us remain actively cognizant of these factors and thoughtfully adjust our pharmacologic interventions to mitigate the collateral damage of these disagreeable effects whenever feasible.*

DM

If every drug in the world were abolished, a physician would still be a useful member of society.
Sir William Withey Gull
(1816-1890; English physician)

✦ The person who takes medicine must recover twice, once from the disease and once from the medicine.

Sir William Osler
(1849-1919; Canadian physician)

✦ Medicine sometimes snatches away health, sometimes gives it.

Ovid
(43 BC-~18 AD; Roman poet)

✦ The worst thing about medicine is that one kind makes another necessary.

Elbert Hubbard
(1856-1915; American writer, artist, & philosopher)

✦ You should treat as many patients as possible with the new drugs while they still have the power to heal.

Armand Trousseau
(1801-1867; French physician)

✦ We are overwhelmed as it is, with an infinite abundance of vaunted medicaments, and here they add another one.

Thomas Sydenham
(1624-1689; English physician)

✦ If you are too fond of new remedies, first you will not cure your patients; secondly, you will have no patients to cure.

Sir Astley Paston Cooper
(1768-1841; English surgeon & anatomist)

✦ Whoever grows angry amid troubles applies a drug worse than the disease and is a physician unskilled about misfortunes.

Sophocles
(~497 BC-405 BC; Greek playwright)

✦ The remedy is often worse than the disease.

Traditional proverb

✦ Poison is in everything, and no thing is without poison. The dosage makes it either a poison or a remedy.

Paracelsus
(1493-1541; Swiss physician)

✦ Poisons and medicine are oftentimes the same substance given with different intents.

Peter Mere Latham
(1789-1875; English physician)

✦ A potent poison becomes the best drug on proper administration. On the contrary, even the best drug becomes a potent poison if used badly.

Charaka
(3rd century BC; Indian physician)

✦ Everything is poisonous, nothing is poisonous, it is all a matter of dose.

Claude Bernard
(1813-1878; French physiologist)

✦ The right dose differentiates a poison from a remedy.

Paracelsus
(1493-1541; Swiss physician)

✦ I confidently affirm that the greater part of those who are supposed to have died of gout, have died of the medicine rather than the disease — a statement in which I am supported by observation.

Thomas Sydenham
(1624-1689; English physician)

✦ I love doctors and hate their medicine.

Walt Whitman
(1819-1892; American writer)

✦ One of the first duties of the physician is to educate the masses not to take medicine.

Sir William Osler
(1849-1919; Canadian physician)

✦ He's the best physician that knows the worthlessness of most medicines.

Benjamin Franklin
(1706-1790; author, inventor,
scientist, politician, & statesman)

✦ It is easy to get a thousand prescriptions, but hard to get one single remedy.

Chinese proverb

✦ Medicines are not meat to live by.

German proverb

✦ Medicine that heals is not always sweet and caring words are not always pleasant.

Tibetan proverb

✦   Medicine cures the man who is fated not to die.

Chinese proverb

Chapter 12

Heed the laws of nature

The physician heals, Nature makes well.
Aristotle
(384 BC-322 BC; Greek philosopher)

● We do not always have the ability or wisdom to alter the natural course of illness and at times we should not impede the natural mechanisms of recovery which are often best left to their own devices with a tincture of time. While the following quotations may seem like overarching naturalistic ideals, we should nevertheless heed their foundational truths.

The natural course of some disease processes and the intangible processes of healing in many instances remain poorly understood. In many cases we have yet to unlock these elusive mechanisms. Nevertheless, under certain clinical circumstances, we should allow these processes to evolve without undue iatrogenic interference. Without undue interference from our inherent meddlesome tendencies as physicians, these natural factors can accomplish much more for our patients than we could ever hope to replicate.

To interfere with the autonomous healing mechanisms and wonders of the natural world would be synonymous with embracing an antithetic view of the Hippocratic Oath as this would translate into doing harm rather than doing good. We as physicians should dutifully execute our work but remember that it is God and nature that ultimately produce the healing.

DM

Nature, time and patience are three great physicians.
Henry George Bohn
(1796-1884; British publisher)

✦ The physician is only nature's assistant.

Galen
(129 AD-210 AD; Greek physician & philosopher)

✦ Nature makes penicillin; I just found it.

Alexander Fleming
(1881-1955; Scottish physician,
microbiologist, & pharmacologist)

✦ Fever itself is Nature's instrument.

Thomas Sydenham
(1624-1689; English physician)

✦ The book of Nature is that which the physician must read; and to do so he must walk over the leaves.

Paracelsus
(1493-1541; Swiss physician)

✦ Healing, Papa would tell me, is not a science, but the intuitive art of wooing Nature.

Wystan Hugh Auden
(1907-1973; English-American poet)

✦ Nature is nowhere accustomed more openly to display her secret mysteries than in cases where she shows tracings of her workings apart from the beaten paths; nor is there any better way to advance the proper practice of medicine than to give our minds to the discovery of the usual law of nature, by careful investigation of cases of rarer forms of disease.

William Harvey
(1578-1657; English physician)

✦ We must alter theory to adapt it to nature, but not nature to adapt it to theory.

Claude Bernard
(1813-1878; French physiologist)

✦ The art of medicine consists of amusing the patient while nature cures the disease.

Francois-Marie Arouet, known
by his nom de plume, Voltaire
(1694-1778; French writer & philosopher)

✦ Here's good advice for practice: go into partnership with nature; she does more than half the work and asks none of the fee.

Martin H. Fischer
(1879-1962; German-American physician & author)

✦ The doctor is the servant and the interpreter of nature. Whatever he thinks or does, if he follows not in nature's footsteps he will never be able to control her.

Giorgio Baglivi
(1668-1707; Italian physician)

✦ The art of healing comes from nature, not from the
physician. Therefore the physician must start from
nature, with an open mind.

Paracelsus
(1493-1541; Swiss physician)

✦ Only by understanding the wisdom of natural foods and
their effects on the body, shall we attain mastery of
disease and pain, which shall enable us to relieve the
burden of mankind.

William Harvey
(1578-1657; English physician)

✦ Time is generally the best doctor.

Ovid
(43 BC-~18 AD; Roman poet)

✦ To do nothing is sometimes a good remedy.

Hippocrates
(460 BC-370 BC; Greek physician)

✦ When you do not know the nature of the malady, leave it to nature; do not strive to hasten matters. For either nature will bring about the cure or it will itself reveal clearly what the malady really is.

Avicenna
(980 AD-1037 AD; Persian physician)

✦ When you are called to a sick man, be sure you know what the matter is — if you do not know, nature can do a great deal better than you can guess.

Nicholas de Belleville
(1753-1831; French physician)

✦ Once a disease has entered the body, all parts which are healthy must fight it: not one alone, but all. Because a disease might mean their common death. Nature knows this; and Nature attacks the disease with whatever help she can muster.

Paracelsus
(1493-1541; Swiss physician)

✦ The generality have considered that disease is but a confused and disordered effort in Nature, thrown down from her proper state, and defending herself in vain.

Thomas Sydenham
(1624-1689; English physician)

_____

✦ The deviation of man from the state in which he was originally placed by nature seems to have proved to him a prolific source of diseases.

Edward Jenner
(1749-1823; English physician)

_____

✦ A certain author defines a doctor to be a man who writes prescriptions till the patient either dies or is cured by nature.

Peter Shaw
(1694-1763; English physician & author)

_____

✦ In a large proportion of the cases treated by allopathic physicians, the disease is cured by nature and not by them. ...in a lesser, but still not in a small proportion, the disease is cured by nature, in spite of them...

Sir John Forbes
(1787-1861; Scottish physician)

✦ Though the doctors treated him, let his blood, and gave him medications to drink, he nevertheless recovered.

Leo Tolstoy
(1828-1910; Russian author)

✦ Remedies act best when there is a tendency to get well.

Sir William Withey Gull
(1816-1890; English physician)

✦   So many come to the sickroom thinking of themselves as
    men of science fighting disease and not as healers with a
    little knowledge helping nature to get a sick man well.

Auckland Geddes
(1879-1954; British academic, soldier, & diplomat)

―――――――――――――――――――

✦   All that man needs for health and healing has been
    provided by God in nature, the challenge of science is to
    find it.

Paracelsus
(1493-1541; Swiss physician)

―――――――――――――――――――

Chapter 13

Prevention: the best medicine

He who cures a disease may be the skillfullest, but he that
prevents it is the safest physician.

Thomas Fuller

(1608-1661; English author)

⬤ In centuries past, long before the current era of
healthcare, physicians, scientists, and philosophers alike
astutely recognized the value of preventative medicine. This
precept endures as an unbelievably important facet of medical
practice in the contemporary era as well. Removing a small

adenomatous polyp via a screening colonoscopy to thwart the development of a colonic adenocarcinoma is a much better option and much more appealing for a patient than undergoing an oncologic segmental colectomy and hepatic metastectomy, if not worse... Wouldn't you agree?

DM

The aim of medicine is to prevent disease and prolong life, the ideal of medicine is to eliminate the need of a physician.
William James Mayo
(1861-1939; American physician)

✦ The greatest medicine of all is teaching people how not to need it.

Hippocrates
(460 BC-370 BC; Greek physician)

✦ Health is not valued till sickness comes.

Thomas Fuller
(1608-1661; English author)

✦ An ounce of prevention is worth a pound of cure.

Benjamin Franklin
(1706-1790; author, inventor,
scientist, politician, & statesman)

✦   A physician who fails to enter the body of a patient with
the lamp of knowledge and understanding can never treat
diseases. He should first study all the factors, including
environment, which influence a patient's disease, and then
prescribe treatment. It is more important to prevent the
occurrence of disease than to seek a cure.

Charaka
(3rd century BC; Indian physician)

✦   The doctor of the future will give no medication, but will
interest his patients in the care of the human frame, in
diet and in the cause and prevention of disease.

Thomas Edison
(1847-1931; American inventor)

✦   Moderate labor of the body conduces to the preservation
of health, and cures many initial diseases.

William Harvey
(1578-1657; English physician)

✦ Walking is man's best medicine.

Hippocrates
(460 BC-370 BC; Greek physician)

✦ Temperance and labor are the two best physicians of man; labor sharpens the appetite, and temperance prevents from indulging to excess.

Jean-Jacques Rousseau
(1712-1778; Swiss writer & philosopher)

✦ Good for the body is the work of the body, and good for the soul is the work of the soul, and good for either is the work of the other.

Henry David Thoreau
(1817-1862; American writer & philosopher)

✦ The superior doctor prevents sickness; the mediocre doctor attends to impending sickness; the inferior doctor treats actual sickness.

Chinese proverb

✦ Nine times out of ten a case seen early is a case half-cured.

Woods Hutchinson
(1862-1930; English physician)

✦ Early, not late remedies are the most effective.

Latin proverb

✦ Before thirty, men seek disease; after thirty, diseases seek men.

Chinese proverb

✦ A man is as old as his arteries.

Thomas Sydenham
(1624-1689; English physician)

✦ The doctor of the future will give no medicine, but will involve the patient in the proper use of food, fresh air and exercise.

Thomas Edison
(1847-1931; American inventor)

Part III

PHILOSOPHIC INSPIRATION & WORDS TO LIVE BY

Be calm and strong and patient. Meet failure and disappointment with courage. Rise superior to the trials of life, and never give in to hopelessness or despair. In danger, in adversity, cling to your principles and ideals. Aequanimitas!

Sir William Osler

(1849-1919; Canadian physician)

Chapter 14

Pave your professional path for success & value

Real success requires respect for and faithfulness to the highest human values — honesty, integrity, self-discipline, dignity, compassion, humility, courage, personal responsibility, courtesy, and human service.

Michael E. DeBakey

(1908-2008; American cardiovascular surgeon)

⬤ *Successful, productive, and being an individual of value — we all strive to adorn our careers, professional lives, and personal lives with these laudable qualities, don't we? Well,* how does one craft and employ such a plan to become successful and to be of value?

First, you must convince yourself that you can be successful. It must all start there — between your own two ears. Per Sir William Osler, *"The very first step towards success in any occupation is to become interested in it."*

Secondly, you must put in the effort — hard work — and that effort must be sustained. As Winston Churchill noted, *"Continuous effort — not strength or intelligence — is the key to unlocking our potential."*

While being successful is a highly sought after and coveted quality, ultimately, one should aim to see past his or her own successes and heed the sage wisdom of Albert Einstein, *"Strive not to be a success, but rather to be of value."*

Akin to maintaining your own physical health and vitality, being successful and being an individual who lends value to others is truly a lifestyle choice. It is not a character trait that turns on and off and it is not a genetic mechanism that expresses variable penetrance. While this notion may at times be actively or passively rattling around in your head-space, the torch of success and value will remain perpetually aflame if this is something you wholly commit yourself to pursuing.

Aristotle suggested that, "The greatest virtues are those which are most useful to other persons," and Ralph Waldo Emerson echoed this sentiment in saying, "To know even one life has breathed easier because you have lived. This is to have succeeded."

We all have our own individual ideas and definitions of what success should be; however, shouldn't personal success be the penultimate goal that stands second behind our journey to be of true value to society and to others as we carry out our humble service as physicians?

DM

The promises of this world are, for the most part, vain phantoms; and to confide in one's self, and become something of worth and value is the best and safest course.

Michelangelo
(1475-1564; Italian Renaissance man)

✦ Aim above morality. Be not simply good, be good for something.

Henry David Thoreau
(1817-1862; American writer & philosopher)

✦ We make a living by what we get, but we make a life by what we give.

Winston Churchill
(1874-1965; soldier, writer, &
Prime Minister of the United Kingdom)

✦ The world owes nothing to any man, but every man owes something to the world.

Thomas Edison
(1847-1931; American inventor)

✦ The noblest question in the world is: "what good may I do in it?"

Benjamin Franklin
(1706-1790; author, inventor,
scientist, politician, & statesman)

✦ One person can make a difference, and everyone should try.

John F. Kennedy
(1917-1963; 35th President of the United States)

✦ Throw away all ambition beyond that of doing the day's work well. The travelers on the road to success live in the present, heedless of taking thought for the morrow. Live neither in the past nor in the future, but let each day's work absorb your entire energies, and satisfy your wildest ambition.

Sir William Osler
(1849-1919; Canadian physician)

✦ Any man's life will be filled with constant and unexpected encouragement if he makes up his mind to do his level best each day.

Booker T. Washington
(1856-1915; American educator,
author, & presidential advisor)

✦ I have simply tried to do what seemed best each day, as each day came.

Abraham Lincoln
(1809-1865; American statesman, lawyer,
& 16th President of the United States)

✦ I learned this, at least, by my experiment; that if one advances confidently in the direction of his dreams, and endeavors to live the life which he has imagined, he will meet with a success unexpected in common hours.

Henry David Thoreau
(1817-1862; American writer & philosopher)

✦ There is no passion in life to be found playing small — in settling for a life that is less than the one you are capable of living.

Nelson Mandela
(1918-2013; South African anti-apartheid revolutionary,
political leader, & President of South Africa)

✦ I have discovered in life that there are ways of getting almost anywhere you want to go, if you really want to go.

Langston Hughes
(1902-1967; American writer)

✦ If you want to succeed you should strike out on new paths, rather than travel the worn paths of accepted success.

John D. Rockefeller
(1839-1937; American businessman & philanthropist)

✦ If my efforts have led to greater success than usual, this is due, I believe, to the fact that during my wanderings in the field of medicine, I have strayed onto paths where the gold was still lying by the wayside. It takes a little luck to be able to distinguish gold from dross, but that is all.

Robert Koch
(1843-1910; German physician & microbiologist)

✦ Do not go where the path may lead, go instead where there is no path and leave a trail.

Ralph Waldo Emerson
(1803-1882; American writer & philosopher)

✦ People are not remembered by how few times they fail, but by how often they succeed. Every wrong step is another step forward

Thomas Edison
(1847-1931; American inventor)

✦ Try and fail, but don't fail to try.

John Quincy Adams
(1767-1848; American statesman, diplomat,
& 6th President of the United States)

✦ Only those who dare to fail greatly can ever achieve greatly.

Robert F. Kennedy
(1925-1968; American politician, lawyer,
& 64th United States Attorney General)

✦ Success is going from failure to failure without losing your enthusiasm.

Winston Churchill
(1874-1965; soldier, writer, &
Prime Minister of the United Kingdom)

✦ A person who never made a mistake never tried anything new.

Albert Einstein
(1879-1955; German physicist)

✦ The man who does things makes many mistakes, but he never makes the biggest mistake of all — doing nothing.

Benjamin Franklin
(1706-1790; author, inventor,
scientist, politician, & statesman)

✦ It is hard to fail, but it is worse never to have tried to succeed.

Theodore Roosevelt
(1858-1919; American statesman, politician, conservationist,
naturalist, writer & 26th President of the United States)

✦ To succeed, jump as quickly at opportunities as you do at conclusions.

Benjamin Franklin
(1706-1790; author, inventor,
scientist, politician, & statesman)

✦ Enthusiasm is the mother of effort, and without it nothing great was ever achieved.

Ralph Waldo Emerson
(1803-1882; American writer & philosopher)

✦ Intelligence without ambition is a bird without wings.

Salvador Dali
(1904-1989; Spanish artist)

✦ By improving yourself, the world is made better. Be not afraid of growing too slowly. Be afraid only of standing still.

Benjamin Franklin
(1706-1790; author, inventor,
scientist, politician, & statesman)

✦ The minds that rise and become really great are never self-satisfied, but still continue to strive.

Claude Bernard
(1813-1878; French physiologist)

✦ The three great essentials to achieve anything worthwhile are: hard work, stick-to-itiveness, and common sense.

Thomas Edison
(1847-1931; American inventor)

✦ Change is the only constant in life. One's ability to adapt to those changes will determine your success in life.

Benjamin Franklin
(1706-1790; author, inventor,
scientist, politician, & statesman)

✦ The will to win, the desire to succeed, the urge to reach your full potential… these are the keys that will unlock the door to personal excellence.

Confucius
(551 BC-479 BC; Chinese philosopher)

✦ Chance favors the prepared mind.

Louis Pasteur
(1822-1895; French biologist, chemist, & microbiologist)

✦ The unprepared mind cannot see the outstretched hand of opportunity.

Alexander Fleming
(1881-1955; Scottish physician,
microbiologist, & pharmacologist)

✦ There is no short cut to achievement. Life requires
thorough preparation — veneer isn't worth anything.

George Washington Carver
(1864-1943; American scientist & inventor)

✦ When schemes are laid in advance, it is surprising how
often the circumstances will fit in with them.

Sir William Osler
(1849-1919; Canadian physician)

✦ I have been impressed with the urgency of doing.
Knowing is not enough; we must apply. Being willing is
not enough; we must do.

Leonardo da Vinci
(1452-1519; Italian Renaissance man)

✦ If others would think as hard as I did, then they would
get similar results.

Sir Isaac Newton
(1643-1727; English mathematician,
physicist, astronomer, theologian, & author)

✦ There is no substitute for hard work.

Thomas Edison
(1847-1931; American inventor)

✦ I find the harder I work, the more luck I seem to have.

Thomas Jefferson
(1743-1826; American statesman, diplomat, lawyer,
architect, & 3rd President of the United States)

✦ If I am anything, which I highly doubt, I have made myself so by hard work.

Sir Isaac Newton
(1643-1727; English mathematician,
physicist, astronomer, theologian, & author)

✦ Genius is one percent inspiration and ninety-nine percent perspiration.

Thomas Edison
(1847-1931; American inventor)

✦ Far and away the best prize that life has to offer is the chance to work hard at work worth doing.

Theodore Roosevelt
(1858-1919; American statesman, politician, conservationist,
naturalist, writer & 26th President of the United States)

✦ My powers are ordinary. Only my application brings me success.

Sir Isaac Newton
(1643-1727; English mathematician,
physicist, astronomer, theologian, & author)

✦ Success is based on imagination plus ambition and the will to work.

Thomas Edison
(1847-1931; American inventor)

✦ I still take failure very seriously, but I've found that the
   only way I could overcome the feeling is to keep on
   working, and trying to benefit from failures or
   disappointments. There are always some lessons to be
   learned. So I keep on working.

Michael E. DeBakey
(1908-2008; American cardiovascular surgeon)

_____

Chapter 15

Courage, persistence, resilience, & perseverance

Life is not easy for any of us. But what of that? We must have perseverance and above all confidence in ourselves. We must believe that we are gifted for something, and that this thing, at whatever cost, must be attained.

Marie Curie
(1867-1934; Polish chemist & physicist)

● *Courage, persistence, resilience, and perseverance —
these characteristics must be summoned by all healthcare
professionals as we navigate clinical challenges as well as
surmount non-clinical obstacles throughout our careers.*

139

Challenges will assuredly be met along the clinical road of healing, in our personal lives, and in our endeavors to advance medical science and technology.

Setbacks, unforeseen hazards, and missteps are inevitable. As we intercept these obstacles that are inherent to the practice of medicine, they can be dealt with directly as they are encountered or they can be carried around as a chip on one's weary shoulders. The perseverance and resilience mustered during difficult times can define one's character as an individual who triumphs in the face of adversity or as an individual who surrenders to the challenge. More elegantly stated, per the wise words of Washington Irving, "Little minds are tamed and subdued by misfortune; but great minds rise above it."

At times, having the will and courage to take the initial leap of faith in tackling a difficult problem can be the most taxing and time-consuming maneuver. When it seems that rock-bottom is looming ever nearer, mustering the grit to ignite a burning drive to keep moving forward and to never accept defeat demonstrates true courage and character. The problem encountered that is triaged as another setback just may contain the answer you are searching for if you look closely enough.

Ralph Waldo Emerson noted that, "All great masters are chiefly distinguished by the power of adding a second, a third, and perhaps a fourth step in a continuous line. Many a man had taken the first step. With every additional step you enhance immensely the value of your first."

Sometimes we have to remind ourselves to take one more step. Take one more step and keep going. That next step forward just may end up being the prevailing stride that propels you across the finish line or reveals the solution to a problem that you have been earnestly searching for.

Allow the following words of wisdom, from some of the greatest minds throughout history, guide your quest to be successful and to be of value despite the stumbles and failures that will inevitably befall your path along the way.

If what you pursue is true and just, if you never give up and never quit, your dreams and desires will materialize into reality.

DM

Twenty years from now you will be more disappointed by the things that you didn't do than by the ones you did do, so throw off the bowlines, sail away from safe harbor, catch the trade winds in your sails. Explore, Dream, Discover.

Mark Twain
(1835-1910; American writer)

✦ Courage and perseverance have a magical talisman, before which difficulties disappear and obstacles vanish into air.

John Quincy Adams
(1767-1848; American statesman, diplomat,
& 6th President of the United States)

_____

✦ Success is not final, failure is not fatal: it is the courage to continue that counts.

Winston Churchill
(1874-1965; soldier, writer, &
Prime Minister of the United Kingdom)

_____

✦ There is hope in dreams, imagination, and in the courage of those who wish to make those dreams a reality.

Jonas Salk
(1914-1995; American medical researcher & virologist)

_____

✦ Whatever you can do, or dream you can, begin it.
Boldness has genius, power and magic in it.

Johann Wolfgang von Goethe
(1749-1832; German writer & statesman)

✦ No great discovery was ever made without a bold guess.

Sir Isaac Newton
(1643-1727; English mathematician,
physicist, astronomer, theologian, & author)

✦ One man with courage makes a majority.

Andrew Jackson
(1767-1845; soldier & 7th President of the United States)

✦ You can never cross the ocean until you have the courage
to lose sight of the shore.

Christopher Columbus
(1451-1506; Italian explorer)

✦ I learned that courage was not the absence of fear, but the triumph over it. The brave man is not he who does not feel afraid, but he who conquers that fear.

Nelson Mandela
(1918-2013; South African anti-apartheid revolutionary,
political leader, & President of South Africa)

✦ Courage is a kind of salvation.

Plato
(~428 BC-~347 BC; Greek philosopher)

✦ Risks, I like to say, always pay off. You learn what to do, or what not to do.

Jonas Salk
(1914-1995; American medical researcher & virologist)

✦ When entering on new ground we must not be afraid to express even risky ideas so as to stimulate research in all directions. As Priestley put it, we must not remain inactive through false modesty based on fear of being mistaken.

Claude Bernard
(1813-1878; French physiologist)

✦ Take the first step in faith. You don't have to see the whole staircase. Just take the first step.

Martin Luther King, Jr.
(1929-1968; American Baptist minister & civil rights leader)

✦ The most difficult thing is the decision to act, the rest is merely tenacity.

Amelia Earhart
(1897-1937; American aviation pioneer)

✦ Take time to deliberate; but when the time for action arrives, stop thinking and go in.

Andrew Jackson
(1767-1845; soldier & 7th President of the United States)

✦ The best way out is always through.

Robert Frost
(1874-1963; American poet)

✦ *Aut inveniam viam aut faciam* — I shall either find a way or make one.

Hannibal
(247 BC-~181 BC; Carthaginian statesman and general)

✦ The capacity of man himself is only revealed when, under stress and responsibility, he breaks through his educational shell, and he may then be a splendid surprise to himself no less than to this teachers.

Harvey Cushing
(1869-1939; American neurosurgeon & writer)

✦ Falling down is not a failure. Failure comes when you stay where you have fallen.

Socrates
(470 BC-399 BC; Greek philosopher)

✦ Develop success from failures. Discouragement and failure are two of the surest stepping stones to success.

Dale Carnegie
(1888-1955; American writer)

✦ There is no such thing as failure, there's just giving up too soon.

Jonas Salk
(1914-1995; American medical researcher & virologist)

✦ A diamond is a piece of coal that stuck to the job.

Thomas Edison
(1847-1931; American inventor)

✦ Never discourage anyone who continually makes progress, no matter how slow... even if that someone is yourself!

Plato
(~428 BC-~347 BC; Greek philosopher)

✦ If you can't fly then run, if you can't run then walk, if you can't walk then crawl, but whatever you do you have to keep moving forward.

Martin Luther King, Jr.
(1929-1968; American Baptist minister & civil rights leader)

✦ It does not matter how slowly you go as long as you do not stop.

Confucius
(551 BC-479 BC; Chinese philosopher)

✦ Energy and persistence conquer all things.

Benjamin Franklin
(1706-1790; author, inventor, scientist, politician, & statesman)

✦ If the wind will not serve, take to the oars.

Latin proverb

_____

✦ It is not the strongest or the most intelligent who will survive but those who can best manage change.

Charles Darwin
(1809-1882; English naturalist & biologist)

_____

✦ Strength does not come from physical capacity. It comes from an indomitable will.

Mahatma Gandhi
(1869-1948; Indian activist)

_____

✦ Everybody's human — everybody makes mistakes. If you laugh it off and keep going and try to give it your best the next time around, people respect that.

Benjamin Franklin
(1706-1790; author, inventor,
scientist, politician, & statesman)

_____

✦ I was taught that the way of progress was neither swift nor easy.

Marie Curie
(1867-1934; Polish chemist & physicist)

✦ Many of life's failures are people who did not realize how close they were to success when they gave up.

Thomas Edison
(1847-1931; American inventor)

✦ A man without persistence will never make a good shaman or a good physician.

Confucius
(551 BC-479 BC; Chinese philosopher)

✦ If I have ever made any valuable discoveries, it has been due more to patient attention, than to any other talent.

Sir Isaac Newton
(1643-1727; English mathematician,
physicist, astronomer, theologian, & author)

✦ Genius is nothing but a greater aptitude for patience.

Benjamin Franklin
(1706-1790; author, inventor,
scientist, politician, & statesman)

✦ The trouble with most people is that they quit before they start.

Thomas Edison
(1847-1931; American inventor)

✦ Whenever ideas fail, men invent words.

Martin H. Fischer
(1879-1962; German-American physician & author)

✦ Our greatest weakness lies in giving up. The most certain way to succeed is always to try just one more time.

Thomas Edison
(1847-1931; American inventor)

✦ In the middle of difficulty lies an opportunity.

Albert Einstein
(1879-1955; German physicist)

✦ Defeat is simply a signal to press onward.

Helen Keller
(1880-1968; American author)

✦ If there is no struggle there is no progress.

Frederick Douglass
(1818-1895; American abolitionist, writer, & statesman)

✦ What seems to us as bitter trials are often blessings in disguise.

Oscar Wilde
(1854-1900; Irish poet & playwright)

✦ You measure the size of the accomplishment by the obstacles you had to overcome to reach your goals.

Booker T. Washington
(1856-1915; American educator,
author, & presidential advisor)

✦ The harder the conflict, the greater the triumph.

George Washington
(1732-1799; military general &
1st President of the United States)

✦ Be courageous! Have faith! Go forward.

Thomas Edison
(1847-1931; American inventor)

✦ Action creates its own courage and courage is as contagious as fear. You must do the thing you think you cannot do.

Eleanor Roosevelt
(1884-1962; First Lady of the United States)

Chapter 16

Be humble & have humility

Acquire the art of detachment, the virtue of method, and the quality of thoroughness, but above all the grace of humility.

Sir William Osler

(1849-1919; Canadian physician)

Being humble and possessing a healthy store of readily accessible humility are key pillars of being a well-conditioned and adaptable physician. None of us are perfect. We are fallible and our noble profession is an imperfect art. The important thing about this universally fallible nature of our chosen profession is simply to acknowledge this fact and admit to it. Otherwise, without acknowledgement of our own shortcomings, there is no room for growth and improvement. Be humble and allow humility in your own personal and professional imperfections to invigorate your drive to improve, to get better, and to push yourself further.

When a mistake occurs, have the mental fortitude to take ownership of the situation without equivocation and resolve to correct these inevitable missteps through hard work, discipline, and most importantly of all — teamwork. By exercising humility in these circumstances you will thus demonstrate how to be a humble and respected leader. As leaders of healthcare teams, we should not covet praise nor reward. When your team is successful give credit to those who have earned it and where credit is justly due.

Be cognizant of too hastily eschewing opportunities or relationships for growth that you believe are not worth your time or are below your station. There are opportunities for growth and progress in everything if we take the time to look deep enough. We should all remain self-aware of our innate egotistical propensities and seek to limit our self-absorbed and

myopic tendencies, lest we risk neglecting valuable
opportunities when they present themselves.

This particular topic may seem trivial or impractical to some;
however, I don't believe the highly esteemed individuals quoted
below would have counseled us in the matter if it wasn't
important...

DM

After all we are merely the servants of the public, in spite of
our MDs and our hospital appointments.
Sir Henry Howarth Bashford
(1880-1961; English physician & author)

✦ The great doctors all got their education off dirt pavements and poverty — not marble floors and foundations.

Martin H. Fischer
(1879-1962; German-American physician & author)

✦ The more fashionable doctors in Italy, began to delegate to slaves the manual attentions they deemed necessary for their patients... that the art of medicine went to ruin.

Andreas Vesalius
(1514-1564; Flemish anatomist & physician)

✦ A man of very moderate ability may be a good physician, if he devotes himself faithfully to the work.

Oliver Wendell Holmes
(1809-1894; American physician & poet)

✦ Mediocre men often have the most acquired knowledge.
   It is in the darker regions of science that great men are
   recognized; they are marked by ideas which light up
   phenomena hitherto obscure and carry science forward.

Claude Bernard
(1813-1878; French physiologist)

✦ It is sometimes asserted that a surgical operation is or
   should be a work of art... fit to rank with those of the
   painter or sculptor. ...That proposition does not admit of
   discussion. It is a product of the intellectual innocence
   which I think we surgeons may fairly claim to possess,
   and which is happily not inconsistent with a quite
   adequate worldly wisdom.

Wilfred Trotter
(1872-1939; English surgeon)

✦ I would like to see the day when somebody would be
   appointed surgeon somewhere who had no hands, for the
   operative part is the least part of the work.

Harvey Cushing
(1869-1939; American neurosurgeon & writer)

✦ We doctors have always been a simple trusting folk. Did we not believe Galen implicitly for 1500 years and Hippocrates for more than 2000?

Sir William Osler
(1849-1919; Canadian physician)

✦ Science increases our power in proportion as it lowers our pride.

Claude Bernard
(1813-1878; French physiologist)

✦ The fact that your patient gets well does not prove that your diagnosis was correct.

Samuel J. Meltzer
(1851-1920; American physiologist)

✦ The patient has the right to accept your advice or to ignore it.

Martin H. Fischer
(1879-1962; German-American physician & author)

✦ There is no curing a sick man who believes himself to be in health.

Henri Amiel
(1821-1881; Swiss philosopher & poet)

✦ Physicians still retain something of their priestly origin; they would gladly do what they forbid.

Otto von Bismarck
(1815-1898; Prussian statesman)

✦ It is easy for men to give advice, but difficult for one's self to follow; we have an example in physicians: for their patients they order a strict regime, for themselves, on going to bed, they do all that they have forbidden to others.

Philemon
(362 BC-262 BC; Greek poet & playwright)

✦ The person most often late for a doctor's appointment is the doctor himself.

Anonymous

✦ It's amazing what you can accomplish if you do not care who gets the credit.

Harry S. Truman
(1884-1972; 33rd President of the United States)

_____

✦ For having lived long, I have experienced many instances of being obliged, by better information or fuller consideration, to change opinions, even on important subjects, which I once thought right but found to be otherwise.

Benjamin Franklin
(1706-1790; author, inventor,
scientist, politician, & statesman)

_____

✦ I have never met a man so ignorant that I couldn't learn something from him.

Galileo Galilei
(1564-1642; Italian astronomer & physicist)

_____

✦ In success be moderate. Humility makes great men twice
honourable.

Benjamin Franklin
(1706-1790; author, inventor,
scientist, politician, & statesman)

✦ Humility leads to the highest distinction, because it leads
to self-improvement.

Sir Benjamin Collins Brodie
(1783-1862; English physiologist & surgeon)

✦ How few there are who have courage enough to own
their faults, or resolution enough to mend them.

Benjamin Franklin
(1706-1790; author, inventor,
scientist, politician, & statesman)

✦   Cultivate the habit of being grateful for every good thing
     that comes to you, and to give thanks continuously. And
     because all things have contributed to your advancement,
     you should include all things in your gratitude.

                                              Ralph Waldo Emerson
                            (1803-1882; American writer & philosopher)

_____

Chapter 17

Uphold integrity; impugn arrogance, conceit, ignorance, & excuses

The only thing more dangerous than ignorance is arrogance.
Albert Einstein
(1879-1955; German physicist)

● Along the same lines as being humble and having humility, we must be keenly aware of, and not be blinded by, our own ignorance despite an inherently human and egotistical apprehension of doing so. After all, isn't blatant dismissal of our own ignorance simply a manifestation of arrogance and conceit? Doesn't dismissal of our own ignorance, for fear of being labeled "wrong" or thought of as "unwise," ultimately hold us back from moving forward?

Never be afraid to say three of the most terrifying words that exist for any physician to mumble, "I don't know." No one could possibly possess all of the answers to the infinite number of questions that rest beneath the vast umbrella of medical science. Move past the catatonia evoking and paralyzing fear of uttering this short phrase. Per the historic words of Maimonides, "Teach thy tongue to say, 'I don't know,' and thou shalt progress."

Honesty and integrity as well as humble admission of what we don't know, so we may improve, will be among the ultimate virtues upon which one's character is judged. It is just as important to be transparently honest about what we don't know as it is to confidently proclaim to the masses what we do know. In the wise words of Sir William Osler, "To confess ignorance is often wiser than to beat around the bush with a hypothetical diagnosis." Thus, as Shakespeare noted, "No legacy is so rich as honesty."

We are only as good as our last complication and we all make mistakes. There are no absolutes in medicine and we will not *always be right despite our best efforts. Accept this truth as a nidus for growth and impugn excuses related to these inevitabilities. Excuses are just as malignant and insulting, to ourselves and to others, as a refusal to acknowledge our own ignorance. Excuses are nothing more than anchors which arrest progress and inhibit forward inertia. Cut them loose and you will be well on your way. And after all, excuses are like bad opinions. Everybody has one, and no one really wants to hear them.*

DM

We do not know the mode of action of almost all remedies. Why therefore fear to confess our ignorance? In truth, it seems that the words "I do not know" stick in every physician's throat.

Armand Trousseau
(1801-1867; French physician)

✦ Never think that you already know all. However highly you are appraised, always have the courage to say to yourself — I am ignorant.

Ivan Pavlov
(1849-1936; Russian physiologist)

✦ There are only two sorts of doctors: those who practice with their brains, and those who practice with their tongues.

Sir William Osler
(1849-1919; Canadian physician)

✦ The doorstep to the temple of wisdom is a knowledge of our own ignorance.

Benjamin Franklin
(1706-1790; author, inventor,
scientist, politician, & statesman)

✦ I shall not mingle conjectures with certainties.

Sir Isaac Newton
(1643-1727; English mathematician,
physicist, astronomer, theologian, & author)

✦ The greater the ignorance the greater the dogmatism.

Sir William Osler
(1849-1919; Canadian physician)

✦ I am not accustomed to saying anything with certainty
after only one or two observations.

Andreas Vesalius
(1514-1564; Flemish anatomist & physician)

✦ To be uncertain is to be uncomfortable, but to be certain
is to be ridiculous.

Chinese proverb

✦ It is said to await certainty is to await eternity.

Jonas Salk
(1914-1995; American medical researcher & virologist)

✦ There are in fact two things, science and opinion; the former begets knowledge, the latter ignorance.

Hippocrates
(460 BC-370 BC; Greek physician)

✦ The arrival of a good clown exercises a more beneficial influence upon the health of a town than twenty asses laden with drugs.

Thomas Sydenham
(1624-1689; English physician)

✦ Any physician who advertises a positive cure for any disease, who issues nostrum testimonials, who sells his services to a secret remedy, or who diagnoses and treats by mail patients he has never seen, is a quack.

Samuel Hopkins Adams
(1871-1958; American writer)

✦ A half-educated physician is not valuable. He thinks he can cure everything.

Mark Twain
(1835-1910; American writer)

✦ An ignorant doctor is the aide-de-camp of death.

Avicenna
(980 AD-1037 AD; Persian physician)

✦ A smart mother makes often a better diagnosis than a poor doctor.

August Bier
(1861-1949; German surgeon)

✦ Better go without medicine than call in an unskilled physician.

Japanese proverb

✦ Printer's ink, when it spells out a doctor's promise to cure, is one of the subtlest and most dangerous of poisons.

Samuel Hopkins Adams
(1871-1958; American writer)

✦ The only weapon with which the unconscious patient can immediately retaliate upon the incompetent surgeon is hemorrhage.

William Stewart Halsted
(1852-1922; American surgeon)

✦ Imagine for yourself a character, a model personality, whose example you determine to follow, in private as well as in public.

Epictetus
(55 AD-135 AD; Greek philosopher)

✦ Be more concerned with your character than with your reputation. Your character is what you really are while your reputation is merely what others think you are.

Dale Carnegie
(1888-1955; American writer)

✦ Moral excellence comes about as a result of habit. We become just by doing just acts, temperate by doing temperate acts, brave by doing brave acts.

Aristotle
(384 BC-322 BC; Greek philosopher)

✦ In matters of style, swim with the current; in matters of principle, stand like a rock.

Thomas Jefferson
(1743-1826; American statesman, diplomat, lawyer, architect, & 3rd President of the United States)

✦ If it is not right do not do it; if it is not true do not say it.

Marcus Aurelius
(121 AD-180 AD; Roman emperor & philosopher)

_____

✦ A wise man speaks because he has something to say; a fool because he has to say something.

Plato
(~428 BC-~347 BC; Greek philosopher)

_____

✦ Remember not only to say the right thing in the right place, but far more difficult still, to leave unsaid the wrong thing at the tempting moment.

Benjamin Franklin
(1706-1790; author, inventor,
scientist, politician, & statesman)

_____

✦ Courage is what it takes to stand up and speak; courage is also what it takes to sit down and listen.

Winston Churchill
(1874-1965; soldier, writer, &
Prime Minister of the United Kingdom)

✦ The greatest deception men suffer is from their own opinions.

Leonardo da Vinci
(1452-1519; Italian Renaissance man)

✦ Honesty is the first chapter of the book wisdom.

Thomas Jefferson
(1743-1826; American statesman, diplomat, lawyer,
architect, & 3rd President of the United States)

✦ Ninety-nine percent of all failures come from people who have the habit of making excuses.

George Washington Carver
(1864-1943; American scientist & inventor)

✦ Never ruin an apology with an excuse.

Benjamin Franklin
(1706-1790; author, inventor,
scientist, politician, & statesman)

_____

✦ It is wise to direct your anger towards problems — not people; to focus your energies on answers — not excuses.

William Arthur Ward
(1921-1994; American writer)

_____

✦ I never knew a man who was good at making excuses who was good at anything else.

Benjamin Franklin
(1706-1790; author, inventor,
scientist, politician, & statesman)

_____

✦ I attribute my success to this: I never gave or took any excuse.

Florence Nightingale
(1820-1910; English nurse)

_____

Part IV

THE ROAD AHEAD

The glory of medicine is that it is constantly moving forward, that there is always more to learn. The ills of today do not cloud the horizon of tomorrow, but act as a spur to greater effort.

William James Mayo

(1861-1939; American physician)

Chapter 18

Provider wellness

Physician, help yourself: thus help your patient too. Let this be his best help: that he may behold with his eyes the man who heals himself.

Freidrich Neitzsche

(1844-1900; German philosopher & poet)

All physicians, medical professionals, and caretakers must take care of themselves so that they are able to effectively care for others. If we are not good to ourselves, we will lose the capacity to be of benefit to others. If you are ill, *burnt out, or in neglect of your own health and wellbeing, you are doing yourself as well as the patients you are caring for a genuine disservice. You must care for yourself before you can truly care for others.*

DM

That physician will hardly be thought very careful of the health of others who neglects his own.
Galen
(129 AD-210 AD; Greek physician & philosopher)

✦ The physician himself, if sick, actually calls in another physician, knowing that he cannot reason correctly if required to judge his own condition while suffering.

Aristotle
(384 BC-322 BC; Greek philosopher)

✦ A physician who treats himself has a fool for a patient.

Sir William Osler
(1849-1919; Canadian physician)

✦ Always laugh when you can, it is cheap medicine.

Lord Byron
(1788-1824; British poet & politician)

✦ The best way to find yourself is to lose yourself in the service of others.

Mahatma Gandhi
(1869-1948; Indian activist)

✦ The best way to cheer yourself up is to try to cheer somebody else up.

Mark Twain
(1835-1910; American writer)

✦ If you want to lift yourself up, lift up someone else.

Booker T. Washington
(1856-1915; American educator,
author, & presidential advisor)

✦ The young doctor should look about early for an avocation, a pastime, that will take him away from patients, pills, and potions.

Sir William Osler
(1849-1919; Canadian physician)

✦ To do much clear thinking a person must arrange for regular periods of solitude when they can concentrate and indulge the imagination without distraction.

Thomas Edison
(1847-1931; American inventor)

✦ Be faithful in small things because it is in them that your strength lies.

Mother Teresa
(1910-1997; Roman Catholic nun & missionary)

✦ Faith and knowledge lean largely upon each other in the practice of medicine.

Peter Mere Latham
(1789-1875; English physician)

✦ Remember no one can make you feel inferior without your consent.

Eleanor Roosevelt
(1884-1962; First Lady of the United States)

✦ It is not living that matters, but living rightly.

Socrates
(470 BC-399 BC; Greek philosopher)

✦ When you are good to others, you are best to yourself.

Benjamin Franklin
(1706-1790; author, inventor,
scientist, politician, & statesman)

✦ Often a healing takes place in ourselves as we pray for the healing of others.

Michael E. DeBakey
(1908-2008; American cardiovascular surgeon)

✦ I am an optimist. It does not seem too much use being anything else.

Winston Churchill
(1874-1965; soldier, writer, &
Prime Minister of the United Kingdom)

✦ Physician, heal thyself.

John of Kronstadt
(1829-1908; Russian priest)

✦ The weeping philosopher too often impairs his eyesight by his woe, and becomes unable from his tears to see the remedies for the evils which he deplores. Thus it will often be found that the man of no tears is the truest philanthropist, as he is the best physician who wears a cheerful face, even in the worst of cases.

Charles Mackay
(1814-1889; Scottish writer)

Chapter 19

The well-rounded clinician

There are, in truth, no specialties in medicine, since to know fully many of the most important diseases a man must be familiar with their manifestations in many organs.

Sir William Osler
(1849-1919; Canadian physician)

With the continued proliferation of specialization in medicine we have become a diverse group of clinicians who identify with particular specialties and sub-specialties. These concentrated areas of practice and study are extremely important. They are invaluable in providing world-class care in the modern era of medicine. That being said, do not become so entrenched in your own specialty that you do not remain a well-rounded clinician with a sound practical working knowledge of medicine and surgery as a whole.

Take the time as a specialist consultant to share a few pearls of wisdom from your unique breadth of knowledge to whomever may be requesting your clinical expertise. As a specialty physician you may even learn something new from a primary care colleague as you cordially collaborate and care for mutual patients.

Although physicians possess a shared and common medical vernacular, there are unique regional dialects spoken in our respective areas of specialty practice that may not be widely understood. Despite these differences between medical specialties, let us all strive to remain on the same page with the desired end result always being the good of our patients.

We are all on the same team, we are all physicians, and we all started out from the same humble beginnings as we swore the sacred Hippocratic Oath and donned white coats.

DM

It ought... to be understood that no one can be a good physician who has no idea of surgical operations, and that a surgeon is nothing if ignorant of medicine. In a word, one must be familiar with both departments of medicine.

Guido Lanfranchi
(1250-1306; Italian surgeon)

✦ Given one well-trained physician of the highest type and he will do better work for a thousand people than ten specialists.

William James Mayo
(1861-1939; American physician)

✦ Descriptive anatomy is to physiology what geography is to history, and just as it is not enough to know the typography of a country to understand its history, so also it is not enough to know the anatomy of organs to understand their functions.

Claude Bernard
(1813-1878; French physiologist)

✦ The specialist is too commonly hypertrophied in one direction and atrophied in all the rest.

Martin H. Fischer
(1879-1962; German-American physician & author)

✦ The extraordinary development of modern science may be her undoing. Specialism, now a necessity, has fragmented the specialities themselves in a way that makes the outlook hazardous. The workers lose all sense of proportion in a maze of minutiae.

Sir William Osler
(1849-1919; Canadian physician)

✦ A man is a poor physician who has not two or three remedies ready for use in every case of illness.

Asclepiades
(2nd century BC; Greek physician)

✦ The physician who knows only medicine, knows not even medicine.

Mark Twain
(1835-1910; American writer)

✦ That which is used — develops. That which is not used wastes away.

Hippocrates
(460 BC-370 BC; Greek physician)

Chapter 20

We are all scientists

The scope of Medicine is so wide as to give exercise to all the faculties of the mind, and it borrows from the stores of almost every form of human knowledge — it is an epitome of science.

Sir William Withey Gull
(1816-1890; English physician)

● *Whether or not you actively incorporate medical science, academics, or research into your practice is certainly a matter of personal preference. However, without disciplined work in this sector of medicine, further progress in discovering new* technology, therapies, and cures to allay disease and pathology would grind to a screeching halt.

A critical facet of education, research, and experimentation in general, but medical education and medical science in particular, is to know the "why" behind the "what." Knowing the fact, or the "what," is not enough. The "why" must be understood to expound upon the basic factual knowledge of the "what." The "why" and the "what" are not mutually exclusive. They must be united together to extract the maximum amount of information they possess.

More succinctly and elegantly stated per Albert Einstein, "Any fool can know. The point is to understand." If that is not a convincing enough argument, then heed the tutelage of the great Leonardo da Vinci, "It's not enough that you believe what you see. You must also understand what you see."

Therefore, when the "why" behind the "what" cannot be satisfied, we should never sleep content. We should dutifully continue pressing forward in our quest for understanding with unabashed exploitation of all the modern wonders at our disposal until the answers we seek are revealed and awaken us with enlightenment.

DM

Do not become archivists of facts. Try to penetrate to the secret of their occurrence, persistently search for the laws which govern them.

Ivan Pavlov

(1849-1936; Russian physiologist)

✦ In science, the best precept is to alter and exchange our ideas as fast as science moves ahead.

Claude Bernard
(1813-1878; French physiologist)

_____

✦ The natural history of science is the study of the unknown. If you fear it you're not going to study it and you're not going to make any progress.

Michael E. DeBakey
(1908-2008; American cardiovascular surgeon)

_____

✦ We must remain, in a word, in an intellectual disposition which seems paradoxical, but which, in my opinion, represents the true mind of the investigator. We must have a robust faith and yet not believe.

Claude Bernard
(1813-1878; French physiologist)

_____

✦ In writing the history of a disease, every philosophical hypothesis whatsoever, that has previously occupied the mind of the author, should lie in abeyance.

Thomas Sydenham
(1624-1689; English physician)

✦ When we meet a fact which contradicts a prevailing theory, we must accept the fact and abandon the theory, even when the theory is supported by great names and generally accepted.

Claude Bernard
(1813-1878; French physiologist)

✦ All sciences are connected; they lend each other material aid as parts of one great whole, each doing its own work, not for itself alone, but for the other parts; as the eye guides the body and the foot sustains it and leads it from place to place.

Roger Bacon
(~1219-1292; English philosopher)

✦ To be worthy of the name, an experimenter must be at once theorist and practitioner. While he must completely master the art of establishing experimental facts, which are the materials of science, he must also clearly understand the scientific principles which guide his reasoning through the varied experimental study of natural phenomena. We cannot separate these two things: head and hand. An able hand, without a head to direct it, is a blind tool; the head is powerless without its executive hand.

Claude Bernard
(1813-1878; French physiologist)

✦ A scientist who is also a human being cannot rest while knowledge which might be used to reduce suffering rests on the shelf.

Albert Sabin
(1906-1993; Polish-American medical researcher)

✦ Those who do not know the torment of the unknown cannot have the joy of discovery.

Claude Bernard
(1813-1878; French physiologist)

✦ Idiopathic and idiotic have a common stem.

Martin H. Fischer
(1879-1962; German-American physician & author)

✦ We must not forget that when radium was discovered no
one knew that it would prove useful in hospitals. The
work was one of pure science. And this is a proof that
scientific work must not be considered from the point of
view of the direct usefulness of it. It must be done for
itself, for the beauty of science, and then there is always
the chance that a scientific discovery may become like the
radium a benefit for humanity.

Marie Curie
(1867-1934; Polish chemist & physicist)

✦ A man of science rises ever, in seeking truth; and if he
never finds it in its wholeness, he discovers nevertheless
very significant fragments; and these fragments of
universal truth are precisely what constitutes science.

Claude Bernard
(1813-1878; French physiologist)

✦ Solutions come through evolution. They come through asking the right questions, because the answers pre-exist. It is the questions that we must define and discover. You don't invent the answer — you reveal the answer.

Jonas Salk
(1914-1995; American medical researcher & virologist)

———————————————

✦ Theories are like a stairway; by climbing, science widens its horizon more and more, because theories embody and necessarily include proportionately more facts as they advance.

Claude Bernard
(1813-1878; French physiologist)

———————————————

✦ I do what I feel impelled to do, as an artist would. Scientists function in the same way. I see all these as creative activities, as all part of the process of discovery. Perhaps that's one of the characteristics of what I call the evolvers, any subset of the population who keep things moving in a positive, creative, constructive way, revealing the truth and beauty that exists in life and in nature.

Jonas Salk
(1914-1995; American medical researcher & virologist)

✦   The joy of discovery is certainly the liveliest that the
     mind of man can ever feel.

Claude Bernard
(1813-1878; French physiologist)

✦   Nosology (from the Greek 'nosos', meaning disease, and
     'logos', referring to study) is not a sport for the timid, and
     certainly not for those so scrupulous about rules and
     order that they demand consistency in all things.

Sherwin B. Nuland
(1930-2014; American surgeon & writer)

✦   In a word, I consider hospitals only as the entrance to
     scientific medicine; they are the first field of observation
     which a physician enters; but the true sanctuary of
     medical science is a laboratory; only there can he seek
     explanations of life in the normal and pathological states
     by means of experimental analysis.

Claude Bernard
(1813-1878; French physiologist)

✦ The fundamental activity of medical science is to determine the ultimate causation of disease.

Wilfred Trotter
(1872-1939; English surgeon)

✦ A knowledge of the specific element in disease is the key to medicine.

Armand Trousseau
(1801-1867; French physician)

✦ When a physician is called to a patient, he should decide on the diagnosis, then the prognosis, and then the treatment. ...Physicians must know the evolution of the disease, its duration and gravity in order to predict its course and outcome. Here statistics intervene to guide physicians, by teaching them the proportion of mortal cases, and if observation has also shown that the successful and unsuccessful cases can be recognized by certain signs, then the prognosis is more certain.

Claude Bernard
(1813-1878; French physiologist)

✦ Knowing, henceforth, the physiognomy of the disease when allowed to run its own course, you can, without risk of error, estimate the value of the different medications which have been employed. You will discover which remedies have done no harm, and which have notably curtailed the duration of the disease; and thus for the future you will have a standard by which to measure the value of the medicine which you see employed to counteract the malady in question. What you have done in respect of one disease, you will be able to do in respect of many; and by proceeding in this way you will be able, on sure data, to pass judgment on the treatment pursued by your masters.

Armand Trousseau
(1801-1867; French physician)

✦ I do not... reject the use of statistics in medicine, but I condemn not trying to get beyond them and believing in statistics as the foundation of medical science. ...Statistics... apply only to cases in which the cause of the facts observed is still indeterminate. ...There will always be some indeterminism... in all the sciences, and more in medicine than in any other. But man's intellectual conquest consists in lessening and driving back indeterminism in proportion as he gains ground for determinism by the help of the experimental method.

Claude Bernard
(1813-1878; French physiologist)

✦ It is the weight, not numbers of experiments that is to be regarded.

Sir Isaac Newton
(1643-1727; English mathematician,
physicist, astronomer, theologian, & author)

✦ Keep your analysis pure and virtuous.

Theodore Billroth
(1829-1894; Austrian surgeon)

✦ The true worth of an experimenter consists in his pursuing not only what he seeks in his experiment, but also what he did not seek.

Claude Bernard
(1813-1878; French physiologist)

✦ Consider data without prejudice.

Thomas Edison
(1847-1931; American inventor)

✦ The science of life is a superb and dazzlingly lighted hall which may be reached only by passing through a long and ghastly kitchen.

Claude Bernard
(1813-1878; French physiologist)

✦ The truly scientific mind is altogether unafraid of the new, and while having no mercy for ideas which have served their turn or shown their uselessness, it will not grudge to any unfamiliar conception its moment of full and friendly attention, hoping to expand rather than to minimize what small core of usefulness it may happen to contain.

Wilfred Trotter
(1872-1939; English surgeon)

✦ Our ideas are only intellectual instruments which we use to break into phenomena; we must change them when they have served their purpose, as we change a blunt lancet that we have used long enough.

Claude Bernard
(1813-1878; French physiologist)

_____

✦ It is my earnest desire that some of you should carry on this scientific work and keep for your ambition the determination to make a permanent contribution to science.

Marie Curie
(1867-1934; Polish chemist & physicist)

_____

✦ We achieve more than we know. We know more than we understand. We understand more than we can explain.

Claude Bernard
(1813-1878; French physiologist)

_____

✦ To me there has never been a higher source of earthly honor or distinction than that connected with advances in science.

Sir Isaac Newton
(1643-1727; English mathematician,
physicist, astronomer, theologian, & author)

✦ I think of the need for more wisdom in the world, to deal with the knowledge that we have. At one time we had wisdom, but little knowledge. Now we have a great deal of knowledge, but do we have enough wisdom to deal with that knowledge?

Jonas Salk
(1914-1995; American medical researcher & virologist)

✦ Well-observed facts, though brought to light by passing theories, will never die; they are the material on which alone the house of science will at last be built.

Claude Bernard
(1813-1878; French physiologist)

Chapter 21

The future of medicine

What we know is a drop, what we don't know is an ocean.
Sir Isaac Newton
(1643-1727; English mathematician, physicist,
astronomer, theologian, & author)

⬤ *The following quotes are illustrative of how unbelievably far we have progressed, but are also indicative of our unfettered ability to continue pushing the boundaries of medicine, surgery, and medical science even further. The incredibly vast realm of medicine is a seemingly boundless frontier that could accommodate limitless growth. There are sweeping expanses of medical space and wilderness yet to be explored and that remain untouched and fundamentally misunderstood. Are we still in the embryonic stages of understanding the disciplines of medicine and surgery? Who knows? Dare we venture into the untamed wilds to find out together?*

No matter what corner of medicine you find yourself practicing today, let us all wholeheartedly endeavor to continue advancing the art, science, and philosophy that will sustain the medical practices of tomorrow. Through this effort we can loyally continue upon the age-old quest to abate and eliminate the deleterious effects of illness and injury that befall the revered patients we care for.

Every step forward is progress, no matter how small. There has never been a brighter time in the history of the world to continue pushing the envelope further. Never settle and never stop searching. The answers to our questions patiently lay in wait. They are waiting to be revealed as long as we continue faithfully searching for them...

DM

Study the hindrances, acquaint yourself with the causes which have led up to the disease. Don't guess at them, but know them through and through if you can; and if you do not know them, know that you do not, and still inquire. "Cannot" is a word for the idle, the indifferent, the self-satisfied, but it is not admissible in science. "I do not know" is manly if it does not stop there, but to say "I cannot" is a judgment both entirely illogical, and in itself is as bad as favouring the rest in ignorance.

Sir William Withey Gull
(1816-1890; English physician)

✦ Very many maintain that all we know is still infinitely less than all that still remains unknown.

William Harvey
(1578-1657; English physician)

✦ We don't know a millionth of one percent about anything.

Thomas Edison
(1847-1931; American inventor)

✦ I know not how I seem to others, but to myself I am but a small child wandering upon the vast shores of knowledge, every now and then finding a small bright pebble to content myself with while the vast ocean of undiscovered truth lay before me.

Sir Isaac Newton
(1643-1727; English mathematician,
physicist, astronomer, theologian, & author)

✦ I have often wondered and even laughed at those who fancied that everything had been so consummately and absolutely investigated by an Aristotle or a Galen or some other mighty name, that nothing could by any possibility be added to their knowledge.

William Harvey
(1578-1657; English physician)

✦ If everyone is thinking alike, then no one is thinking.

Benjamin Franklin
(1706-1790; author, inventor,
scientist, politician, & statesman)

✦ We shall have no better conditions in the future if we are satisfied with all those which we have at present.

Thomas Edison
(1847-1931; American inventor)

213

✦ If we cannot heal in one way, we must learn to heal in another.

Sherwin B. Nuland
(1930-2014; American surgeon & writer)

✦ Diagnosis is not the end, but the beginning of practice.

Martin H. Fischer
(1879-1962; German-American physician & author)

✦ Nothing in medicine is so insignificant as to merit attention.

Thomas Sydenham
(1624-1689; English physician)

✦ By the help of microscopes, there is nothing so small, as to escape our inquiry; hence there is a new visible world discovered to the understanding.

Robert Hooke
(1635-1703; English philosopher)

✦ In physiology, as in all other sciences, no discovery is useless, no curiosity misplaced or too ambitious, and we may be certain that every advance achieved in the quest of pure knowledge will sooner or later play its part in the service of man.

Ernest Starling
(1866-1927; British physiologist)

✦ A conclusion is the place where you got tired thinking.

Martin H. Fischer
(1879-1962; German-American physician & author)

✦ Nothing is more dangerous than strict logic — which is not quite sure of its premises. ...From the number and deadliness of the maladies that lie in wait for us we have no logical right to expect to survive; and yet we are here in defiance of logic. Of course, this world is a dangerous place and few of us ever get out of it alive; yet the race goes right on living, somehow, undaunted in spite of the new and terrible diseases that medical science keeps discovering.

Woods Hutchinson
(1862-1930; English physician)

✦ It is a most gratifying sign of the rapid progress of our time that our best text-books become antiquated so quickly.

Theodore Billroth
(1829-1894; Austrian surgeon)

✦ It is possible to create an epidemic of health which is self-organizing and self-propelling.

Jonas Salk
(1914-1995; American medical researcher & virologist)

✦ Medicine, the only profession that labors incessantly to destroy the reason for its own existence.

James Bryce
(1838-1922; English diplomat)

✦ Our profession is the only one which works unceasingly to annihilate itself.

Martin H. Fischer
(1879-1962; German-American physician & author)

✦ In my view, art and the approach to life through art,
   using it as a vehicle for education and even for doing
   science is so vital that it is part of a great new revolution
   that is taking place. I believe we are entering a whole
   new epoch.

Jonas Salk
(1914-1995; American medical researcher & virologist)

✦ A great discovery is a fact whose appearance in science
   gives rise to shining ideas, whose light dispels many
   obscurities and shows us new paths.

Claude Bernard
(1813-1878; French physiologist)

✦ This is perhaps the most beautiful time in human history;
   it is really pregnant with all kinds of creative possibilities
   made possible by science and technology which now
   constitute the slave of man — if man is not enslaved by it.

Jonas Salk
(1914-1995; American medical researcher & virologist)

✦ There are no incurable diseases — only the lack of will.
There are no worthless herbs — only the lack of
knowledge.

Avicenna
(980 AD-1037 AD; Persian physician)

✦ We have merely scratched the surface of the store of
knowledge which will come to us. I believe that we are
now, a-tremble on the verge of vast discoveries —
discoveries so wondrously important they will upset the
present trend of human thought and start it along
completely new lines.

Thomas Edison
(1847-1931; American inventor)

✦ The important thing is not to stop questioning.

Albert Einstein
(1879-1955; German physicist)

✦ To cease to think creatively is to cease to live.

Benjamin Franklin
(1706-1790; author, inventor,
scientist, politician, & statesman)

✦ Nothing in life is to be feared, it is only to be understood. Now is the time to understand more, so that we may fear less.

Marie Curie
(1867-1934; Polish chemist & physicist)

Afterword

Regardless of age, the indelible messages contained within these quotations have preserved their potency and elegantly outline the fundamental truths, grounding roots, and foundational ideals that the practice of medicine has been built upon. It is my feeling that these quotations have a unique ability to evoke powerful emotions within us all as physicians. These precepts, tenets, and ideals possess the energy to enrich our view of medical history as well as inspire us to be the best physicians we can be if taken to heart. Similarly, these thoughts seem to harbor an inimitable capacity to calm the surface of a turbulent clinical sea or to brighten the sometimes-clouded

road of healing during trying times. Call on these pearls of
motivation and wisdom on those days when you find yourself
sorely requiring a healthy dose of personal encouragement.
They will always be relevant and they will always be there
when you need them most.

No matter what undercurrents may have guided you into the
calling of medicine, at some level the reason we all became
physicians is because we have a deeply empathetic view of the
human condition. Is it not? It is my sincere wish that these
poetic ideals related to our healing art, now hopefully in clear
perspective and focus, can be incorporated into your daily
practice and will positively impact patient care and your
medical practice as a whole.

I hope you had as much fun reading this collection as I did in
putting it together. I also hope that one day some of you
reading this book now will be quoted in the future and your
contributions added to the timeless art and science of medicine
and surgery.

Godspeed!

Daniel McMahon, MD